Intoxicating Minds

MAPS OF THE MIND

Steven Rose, General Editor

MAPS OF THE MIND

STEVEN ROSE, GENERAL EDITOR

—

Intoxicating Minds

HOW DRUGS WORK

Ciaran Regan

Columbia University Press

New York

Columbia University Press
Publishers Since 1893
New York   Chichester, West Sussex

Copyright © 2001 Ciaran Regan
First published by Weidenfeld and Nicolson Ltd., London

Library of Congress Cataloging-in-Publication Data
Regan, Ciaran.
Intoxicating minds : how drugs work / Ciaran Regan.
p. cm. — (Maps of the mind)
Includes bibliographical references and index.
ISBN 0-231-12016-8
1. Psychopharmacology.   I. Title.   II. Series.

RM315 .R447 2001
615′.78—dc21
2001–028078

∞

Printed in the United States of America

c 10 9 8 7 6 5 4 3 2 1

For Helen

Contents

Preface and Acknowledgments

This book is intended for anyone who is curious about mind-altering drugs. In offering this view, I must immediately temper its contents with a note of modesty. We really do not know how the mind works, let alone how drugs influence it. But not knowing answers is no reason to avoid thinking about the questions. In seeking possible explanations for how drugs work and how they may influence the mind, we need to think scientifically about drugs, how we relate to them, and if they may be of cultural value. What's needed is a grand excavation of the myths surrounding drugs. This is what *Intoxicating Minds* tries to achieve, for it does not extol or condemn drug use; it simply invites reflection.

Few of the ideas that follow are mine, for I have discovered no new theory about how drugs may influence the mind. What I have done is to select ideas from many disciplines and mold them into a broad concept—to present the facts and to suggest new ideas. The book is not written for the academic, nor is it an attempt to popularize science, for, nowadays, there is little difference between a thoughtful individual and the professional whose expertise is limited to a tightly defined discipline. I hope it will interest the general reader. This means that much is presented in rather simple terms. I hope to have been successful in making the book readable and enjoyable. A list of books is provided at the end for those who may wish to read further on any aspect of the topic.

Many have played a crucial role in forming my ideas on mind-altering drugs. Foremost are my students at University College Dublin, who, perhaps unwittingly, have served to sharpen my ideas on the effects of drugs through years of endless questions. But I must pay tribute to John Marshall, a neuropsychologist, for driving me to study the brain. When I was a young postdoctoral fellow of the European Molecular Biology Organization at the University of Nijmegen, in the Netherlands, interested only in the subtleties of protein chemistry, he forced me to provide biochemical concepts that would account for the emerging idea of brain plasticity. The whole concept has continued to captivate me. I now owe a debt of gratitude to the many students and postdoctoral researchers for their contributions to my research on this subject. But I must especially thank Larry Bacon, Helen Gallagher, and Keith Murphy, who ensured that research continued at University College Dublin during my days of absence while writing this book, for their contributions to its concepts.

Many thanks are due also to those who have commented on earlier versions of the manuscript. These include close colleagues and friends—Alan Baird, Ron Beyma, Alan Keenan, Brian Leonard, Amanda McCann, Martin Murphy, Kathy O'Boyle, Cormac O'Connell, and Veronica Jane O'Mara. Their remarks have improved the manuscript and eliminated many errors. My editors, Peter Tallack at Weidenfeld and Nicolson, Holly Hodder at Columbia University Press, and the series editor Steven Rose were all I could have wanted—exacting perfectionists who demanded clarity—and I am greatly indebted to them.

Finally, I must recognize my younger daughter, Helen, for her unwavering interest in the adventure and utter belief in its completion. Too young to understand or criticize, I hope that one day she will read this book, for it is dedicated to her.

Intoxicating Minds

Mists of the Mind

Intoxicating Minds

This is a book about drugs and how they affect our minds. Since the beginning of recorded history, drugs have been used for pleasure, for the treatment of insanity, and for relief from the mundane—they are a unique characteristic of human life and society. Virtually all of our important social interactions combine drugs that have the potential to alter our recall of events in one way or another. However minimal, these effects alter how we convey and sustain our experiences of the recent past—those memories that ultimately form our mind. Is alcohol used to eliminate memories that separate individuals? Does caffeine enhance sociability, thereby enriching our society through the acceptance and incorporation of diverse individuals and new ideas?

Drugs, such as heroin or cocaine, can create a signal in the brain that indicates, falsely, a feeling of confidence—a huge fitness benefit. This changes behavioral propensities so that drug-seeking predominates and displaces our more adaptive behaviors. But some drugs can also improve adaptation in some circumstances, relieve the symptoms of mental disorders, and induce pleasures that can sometimes be safe. To what extent do these drug-altered states contribute to our survival, and are they culturally valuable?

The brain requires trillions of connections between its billions of nerve cells to function properly. The mere 100,000 genes aligned along our chromosomes are simply insufficient to specify this fantastic connectivity pattern, let alone the modifications required to store information acquired over a lifetime. But the brain is dynamic; it continually reorders the pattern of its nerve cell connections in response to experience, thereby creating the unique nature of every individual in relation to his or her past.

Our memories do not seem to be secured immediately—the hotel room is forgotten by the time the homeward plane has been boarded. But we have no difficulty in remembering the births of our children or how to ride a bicycle. It would seem that memory is initially fragile but with time grows more robust. And if this is true, then the period of memory frailty must surely be exquisitely sensitive to drugs—they must be capable of influencing past events, those experiences that ultimately form our minds.

These are the topics *Intoxicating Minds* strives to address. What I hope will distinguish this book is that it does not fall into any one generic category, for it embraces biology and medicine and sociology and anthropology—all intertwined with stories of scientific and artistic achievement, war and greed, empires and religions, and lessons for our own future.

Storylines

Since prehistory, remembering has rarely been a cerebral exercise alone. Bardic reiteration of epic themes, from Homer's *Iliad* to the peripatetic poetry of Gaelic Ireland or the complex narratives painted on caves or the stress-induced release of adrenaline during oaths, magic, and sacrifices, have all served to ensure the accuracy and continuance of our memories. Commemorative ceremonies are preeminent instances of remembering. The liturgy of the Christian Mass has persisted for nearly two millennia, and during this time it has changed very slowly. It keeps the past in mind through a reenactment of previous events that are central to the belief of the faithful.

But we can also preserve the past deliberately without explicitly representing it in words and images. We may not remember how or when we first learned to swim, but we can keep on swimming successfully, remembering how to do it without any representational activity on our part. In habitual memory the past seems to precipitate in the body. The rehearsing and arousing nature of these ritualized actions appears to reinforce our memory of prior experiences that otherwise might be lost with the passage of time. Memory needs to be reinforced if it is to be retained.

Many communities have incorporated the use of stimulants into these ritual actions and commemorative ceremonies, and, with time, they have evolved from a sacred to secular context. *Coca*, which contains cocaine, provides an interesting example. This stimulant is obtained from the leaves of *Erythroxylum coca*, a shrub that was well established in the eastern highlands of the Andes mountains during the time of the Incas. They venerated coca as a gift from the gods because it could alleviate hunger and renew their vigor. These "coca chewers" were skillful: using either ash or lime juice, they made their saliva more alkaline and so improved delivery of the maximum dose.

The Incas restricted coca to their religious ceremonies and initiation rituals, and used it to produce trance-like states in order to commune with the spirits. It was far too valuable a commodity to be used by the common Indians. But its sacred context quickly became a secular one in the face of the onslaught by Pisarro and his conquistadors. The "commoners" indulged in coca chewing, addiction became widespread, and its use almost banned—until the Spaniards found their slaves worked harder and longer when chewing coca.

Coca was introduced to Europe by the returning conquistadors and became popular as a social drink in the form of an alcoholic beverage known as *Vin Maraini*. It even received an official seal of approval from Pope Leo XIII. It entered the United States as Pemberton's French wine, but, with prohibition in 1919, the wine was removed, replaced with caffeine from kola nuts, and Coca Cola was advertised as the "temperance drink." Eventually, the coca was removed and, with much legal wrangling, the name was saved. By the end of the nineteenth century, however, cocaine had become tremendously popular, as many scientists and physicians, including Sigmund Freud, lauded its properties. By 1885 Parke Davis and Company was manufacturing fifteen different forms of coca and cocaine, including cigarettes, inhalants, and even tooth drops to relieve the discomfort of infant teething. When cocaine was proscribed around 1915, its use eventually became restricted to small groups of avant-garde artists and musicians. But at the beginning of the 1970s an epidemic of cocaine use reemerged. Lime juice was no longer needed: direct delivery to the bloodstream could be achieved by smoking, snorting, or injecting the drug in its pure form.

Not all communities pursue intoxication in this arbitrary and hedonistic fashion. Our assimilation of stimulants such as tea and tobacco, first used in other cultures in sacred and ceremonial settings, has resulted in their being divested of any spiritual significance. Indeed, the fundamental role of these substances is essentially a communal one, namely, that of stimulating sociability. The offering of tea or coffee to friends and strangers alike is a common form of extending hospitality. Nevertheless, they allow differences in social status to be maintained, sometimes by the order in which the participants take the stimulant as well as in the great ingenuity and craftsmanship invested in creating the distinctive equipment that accompanies consumption. In traditional societies such artefacts reveal both the social status of the user and the symbolic importance of the occasion on which they are used. Items from our own culture, such as cut-glass decanters, gold cigarette cases, and porcelain tea sets, hint at the competition for social status that goes on just below the surface of these apparently innocuous customs.

Our culture is embedded with myths and driven by changes that have been attendant on the use of mind-altering drugs. In a sanctuary at Eleusis, near Athens, there was an annual celebration that lasted for over 2,000 years. It symbolized for the Greeks the natural enigma of the changing seasons and the cultivation of grain on which their civilization depended. This fertility cult involved drinking a secret potion called *kykeon* that provided the participants with mystical visions. The potion was prepared from barley infected with the ergot fungus, which contains compounds closely related to LSD. Flying ointments, long associated with European witchcraft folklore, were prepared from plants containing mind-altering agents. In literature many of the sequences written by Lewis Carroll in *Through the Looking Glass*, for example, are an accurate reflection of the effects of ingesting the familiar red mushroom with white spots (*Amanita muscaria*) often illustrated in books of children's fairy tales. The infamous association of French writers and artists known as Le Club des Hachichins included such notables as Victor Hugo, Alexander Dumas Théophile Gautier, and Charles Baudelaire, who extolled the use of cannabis to improve their artistic performance. And in music the Beatles' song "Lucy in the Sky with Diamonds," with its "tangerine trees and marmalade skies," in many ways describes the effects of LSD. Drug use seems to attend many of our cultural advances.

Vade Mecum

As a research scientist, I am interested in the molecular mechanisms we use to process our experiences and render them indelible as long-term memory. This process of memory formation can take days to weeks in animals and even decades in humans; during this period the memory trace remains exquisitely sensitive to the action of drugs. Some drugs improve memory while others eliminate it. But memory is no ordinary faculty. Without memory we cannot adapt to our ever-changing circumstances and would fail to survive in society. Just as society is a form of memory that determines our sense of individuality, it is the landscape of our minds. As Karl Marx put it: "It is not the consciousness of men [*sic*] that determines their being but, on the contrary, their social being that determines their consciousness." The inescapable conclusion, at least for me, is that drug use has the potential to alter the mind and the evolution of societies. That is the conundrum I wish to address in this book.

Undertaking this task has been no easy matter. For example, the classic approach of dealing with drugs in defined categories while hoping that readers will see the obvious trends and links did not appear to be the answer. Many textbooks have adopted this approach and, frankly, have failed to convey the excitement I feel about the role of drugs in society. Such books tend to be dogmatic and operate within the classical constraints of science. Moreover, most of this literature is inaccessible to the general reader because it is expressed in the runic gabble of chemical formulae, mathematical derivations, and terse descriptions of drug effects on the brain. Another approach was necessary.

In the end the approach I adopted for this book was to concentrate on drugs that have made a significant impact on society, those that have been actively sought by humans purely for their mind-altering properties. In other words, the book represents my views on the reciprocal relationships among drugs, behavior, and society. This means that I have paid scant attention to many drugs that alter brain function, such as *general anesthetics* and those used to treat epilepsy, Parkinson's disease, or Alzheimer's disease. This is because I do not view these to be true mind-altering drugs. Rather they are used to control or replace lost function or, in the case of general anaesthetics, to render an individual unconscious in preparation for surgery. Nevertheless, where appropriate, I have made brief comments on how these drugs are believed to be effective.

In addition to the mechanisms by which drugs influence brain function, I will also show that the basic scientific principles, both direct and indirect, have their origins in antiquity. We need to be aware, therefore, of the historical world of societies from which we have evolved. Faithful encoding of memory is critical to our adaptation and survival, and is of central importance to the evolution of society. The book attempts to explain how drug use has evolved to become an integral part of our daily repertoires and the structure of our society. This approach has proved to be invaluable. For example, the development of drugs to treat disorders of the mind, such as schizophrenia and depression, is a Herculean task and one that can only be understood in a historical context. History is not just one fact after another—it has patterns, and the search for their explanation is as productive as it is fascinating.

The first few short chapters are therefore intended to introduce the language of the scientist, to allow you to become familiar with the terms and the concepts we so often bandy about without explanation. These chapters define the nature of drugs, and they explain how drugs influence the workings of the brain and how these actions relate to that elusive concept called the *mind*. With this toolbox in place, I deal with the effects of stimulants, such as caffeine and nicotine, on brain function and explore the reasons and consequences for their sudden assimilation into the culture of Western society in the seventeenth century. Then I discuss the rise and use of more modern stimulants, such as cocaine and ecstasy, and this leads to ideas about the greed for drugs that provide pleasure—how the craving for alcohol or heroin can be attributed to the physical alterations they produce in the brain. This is followed by a short interlude on how we process memory for long-term storage—the molecular mechanisms of memory. That provides a basis for our understanding of how drugs can configure the mind, and it prepares us to comprehend the nature of thought disorder and the therapies used to treat depression and schizophrenia. From there I consider psychedelic drugs from the perspective of their perceived mystical and cosmic properties, an idea which has had such a significant influence on the fabric of our society. The mystical properties of placebos—drugs used to alleviate certain diseases, which in fact are ineffective for those conditions—provide an opportunity to trace how modern medicine and drug therapies emerged from past civilizations that existed in Alexandria and the river valleys of the Nile, Tigris, and Euphrates. The book concludes by considering the physical consequences of our coevolution with drugs and how they have altered the very essence of our being; last, we take a brief glimpse at possible drug therapies for the future.

Matters of Doctrine

Definitional Dilemmas

Consult any textbook of pharmacology and, if lucky, you may be informed that a *drug* is any "chemical that affects living processes." It is more likely that such texts will define *pharmacology* as "the study of the manner in which the function of living systems is affected by chemical agents" and, in so doing, avoid the drug definition issue completely. It would seem that the originators of these texts wish us to conclude that any chemical agent is a drug and that pharmacology describes the physical effects of these chemicals on the body.

The term *pharmacology* stems from the Greek word *pharmakos*. But this also can be interpreted to mean a scapegoat, a person who was sacrificed as a remedy for whatever maladies another person might have been suffering. Alternatively, *pharmakos* can mean a charm, whether healing or poisonous. The dilemma is exemplified by digoxin (Lanoxin), a drug found in the leaves of the purple foxglove (*Digitalis purpurea*), which has a long history of use in the treatment of heart failure. Appropriate doses of digoxin increase heart rate and relieve the associated build-up of tissue fluid; inappropriate doses can be lethal because they generate irregular patterns of heartbeat, which lead to cardiac arrest. Considered in this way, digoxin may be defined as both a drug and a poison.

General *anaesthetics* are a group of chemicals with consequences not unlike those of digoxin. The history of using volatile liquids to render an individual unconscious for the purpose of carrying out surgical procedures is surprisingly recent. In the mid-1800s laughing gas, or nitrous oxide, was popular in fairgrounds because it quickly rendered the unsuspecting individual "drunk," much to the amusement of the onlookers—hence the origin of the term "laughing gas." Ether, another volatile liquid, has similar effects and was used by students to produce states of drunken euphoria at parties that were often referred to as "ether frolics." With increasing amounts of these gases, however, it was noted that users became temporarily unconscious but recovered, relatively unscathed, sometime later. The potential of such chemicals to relieve pain during surgery became obvious, and their effectiveness was first publicly demonstrated at the Massachusetts General Hospital in 1846 during the removal of a tumor from a patient's lower jaw.

While the art of using inhalational anaesthetics for surgery is now routine for many surgical procedures, there is one technical aspect to their use that is not always so obvious: they block our natural reflexes. Initially, we lose our skills of coordination, but as the dose is increased our cardiac and respiratory reflexes become blunted, and this can lead to death if the dose is not carefully controlled. Like digoxin, chemicals can be useful in moderate doses but prove deadly when greater amounts are administered. This is why the *dose-response effect* preoccupies the pharmacologist.

But we must also take into account the drug's effects on the body. When a drug is taken orally, it is absorbed from the stomach or intestine and enters the bloodstream, which carries it to all areas of the body. To enter the bloodstream, the drug must pass through a whole series of barriers—mainly the membranes that surround all cells, including those that form the stomach and intestine, blood vessels, and body tissues. This is why the effects of a drug are more immediate when it is injected directly into the bloodstream. Inhaling a drug like nicotine, or snorting a drug such as cocaine, produces similar rapid effects because the lungs and membranes of the nasal cavity are densely packed with blood vessels through which the drug can gain more direct access to the bloodstream.

Yet not all individuals respond to a drug in the same way. Take alcohol as an example. The sensitivity of individuals to the effects of alcohol varies greatly. Gender is one factor that determines the degree of euphoric and damaging effects produced by alcohol. Women have proportionately more body fat than men, and because alcohol cannot enter fat stores, a higher concentration tends to accumulate in the bloodstream of women, even when the same amount of alcohol is consumed by a man and woman of similar weight. Genetic differences also determine sensitivity to alcohol. Some Asian populations and Native Americans have a reduced ability to eliminate alcohol from the body compared with European populations. This difference is due to variations in the activity of *enzymes* involved in the elimination of alcohol. Enzymes are the catalytic converters of the body—they are proteins that remain unchanged as they convert one biochemical compound into another. In the Asian and Native American populations, the enzymes are less active than in most Europeans. These differences, which are genetic in origin, make certain populations more susceptible to the effects of alcohol.

Once a drug is absorbed into the bloodstream, it must eventually pass through the liver where it may be modified further. This is called the *first-pass effect*, and it usually results in the inactivation and elimination of some of the drug dose. But this step can also result in the activation of certain drugs. *Benzodiazepines* are used to treat anxiety, and many of them are transformed again and again into other active forms as they are recycled through the liver. Nearly all tissues of the body are capable of metabolizing drugs. Parkinson's disease is a movement disorder that arises from the decay of nerve cells in a brain region that controls our motor skills. This disease is treated with levodopa, which is inactive when taken orally but converted into the active form by nerve cells in the brain. In the active form, this drug serves to correct the movement disorder by boosting the action of nerve cells that have not yet degenerated. The first-pass effect may also convert a drug into a toxin. Halothane, for example, is a general anaesthetic gas that can be converted into trifluoroacetic acid, a chemical that can cause significant damage to all tissues of the body.

But drugs are subject to many other definitions. What is the distinction between a food and a drug? Certain vitamins and minerals found in our diet can be isolated and used to control disease—for example, administering vitamin C treats scurvy. There are more subtle aspects, such as the definition of a drug used for medical and nonmedical purposes. Caffeine can be used to treat migraines or simply enjoyed for the stimulant qualities of a cup of coffee. How do we define a drug for therapeutic use rather than recreational use? Cocaine is considered widely to be a recreational drug in spite of the fact that it has therapeutic utility as a local anaesthetic.

Drug use or prohibition seems to be dependent on a tight set of rules that are the laws, customs, and practices operating at a given time and place. Attitudes to nonmedical drugs, such as alcohol and nicotine, vary in different countries. Alcohol was proscribed in the United States during a short period of social disapproval, whereas the Islamic religion totally forbids its use. The unavoidable fact of the matter is that a substance becomes a drug in the pejorative sense when, and only when, interdicted by a law or social norm. One begins to appreciate why the pharmacologist is much happier defining how a drug works than classifying what it may be.

Mind Dust

Drugs that predominantly affect the mind are usually referred to as *psychoactive* drugs. The term *psychoactive* is derived from the Greek word *psyche*, which originally referred to the soul or spirit but in today's usage refers to the mind. Hence the term *psychopharmacology* refers to understanding the influence of drugs on the mind. These drugs have provided some of the most important therapeutic advances in the past fifty years of pharmacology. They have released schizophrenics from the confinement of institutions, provided relief from the otherwise long-lasting pain of depression, and eased the debilitating effects of anxiety. In contrast, the euphoric effects of alcohol, opium, heroin, and morphine have provided relief from pain but have also plagued us with addiction. Yet psychoactive drugs are also recreational: caffeine and nicotine serve to stimulate our mental activity; amphetamine and cocaine make us confident and fearless; and LSD provides awesome and incredible images that relieve the mundane and reveal, for some, a divine knowledge of the inner self.

While the term *psychopharmacology* may appear to be obvious and serve to classify broadly the action of psychoactive drugs, it encompasses a territory that is largely uncharted. Most texts state that LSD is a mind-altering drug or comment that alcohol modifies our state of consciousness without attempting to define the precise nature of the effects that these terms are supposed to describe. This cop-out always reminds me of a story in the book *The Astonishing Hypothesis* in which the author Francis Crick recalls his wife was taught the Roman Catholic catechism by an elderly Irish lady who pronounced the word *being* as "be-in." Although puzzled by the definition of a soul as a living "bean" without a body, his wife kept the worries to herself. To some extent, the same problem exists in the world of psychopharmacology.

Relating mind to brain always brings up the rather thorny issue of consciousness. While we all have a subjective sense of its meaning, an adequate definition of consciousness still eludes us. It seems obvious that awareness must be an important aspect of consciousness. Our level of attentiveness and prior knowledge, as stored in our long-term memories, must also enrich our degree of awareness.

There are many types of awareness, which differ in their degree of complexity. With sensory awareness, for example, we can speak of the ambient temperature through the information conveyed from the temperature sensors in our skin. We tend to speak more or less interchangeably of being aware of states of the world and being aware of the sensations that inform us of those states. Sensory awareness is not an elusive phenomenon: it is sensitive to certain psychoactive drugs. Ingesting small doses of LSD can result in the "seeing" of smells or the "hearing" of colors, an effect known as *synesthesia.* LSD must trigger these nonordinary states of sensory awareness, since it would be a pharmacological fallacy to believe that the drug contains these experiences.

We can also be aware of our inner states. This is a generalized form of awareness that does not necessarily relate to the sensations received from the environment. We can, for example, be aware of a generalized sense of fatigue. We can often experience a prevailing sense of anxiety for no obvious reason. Psychoactive drugs can also influence these generalized states of awareness. Alcohol alleviates anxiety, and cocaine our sense of fatigue.

Cognitive or reflective awareness, however, is more complex. It can involve being unconsciously aware or becoming consciously aware of events that occurred earlier. *Blindsight* is a form of unconscious awareness. The visual cortex is a region at the back of the brain that is involved in the perception of the visual stimuli that make up the images that surround us. Patients with damage to the visual cortex are blind despite the fact that their retina is functionally intact. Nevertheless, such patients can "guess" their location in a given environment with an accuracy greater than random guess work.

There is also awareness of our prior experiences, which is both conscious and unconscious. Damage to a brain region called the *hippocampus* results in amnesia, a complete loss of conscious recall for recent events. Yet such patients often retain an unconscious memory for certain types of skills. When asked to trace the mirror image of a star, for example, they quickly become proficient at the task and retain this aptitude when tested at a later date. It seems that unconscious recall for the task is preserved and associated with brain regions other than the hippocampus, possibly in areas such as the *striatum*, a region that coordinates motor skills. Psychoactive drugs can also discriminate between these two forms of memory. Scopolamine, for example, only blocks recall of conscious memory and has no effect on the unconscious recall of acquired skills.

Suggesting awareness to be synonymous with consciousness is a cheap way of dealing with the conundrum of relating brain to mind. Consciousness is much more: it is the way we deal with the world around us—our relationship to a lover, family member, or culture. We get into difficulties when we try to understand this condition in others. People suffering from depression, for example, describe a feeling of "intense mental pain" that no one but the sufferer can understand, as it is their subjective emotion. I can sense the euphoric effect of alcohol, but I cannot know if my experience is similar to that of others. Consciousness is the very nature of each individual's existence. Yet what we consciously experience is closely related to the activities of the brain, since psychoactive drugs or damage to discrete brain regions can significantly influence it. This suggests that consciousness is not a commodity but a process that allows our brains to report our changing condition to others and ourselves.

3

Making the Mind

Spirits of the Mind

Neural activity in the brain cannot be divorced from the function of its basic units, the *nerve cells* or *neurons*. These are specialized to perform one major job: information transfer. Neurons come in all shapes and sizes and are only obvious when viewed with a microscope. Numerous extensions emanate from the main cell body, which contains the nucleus and its DNA, the string of small molecules called *nucleotides*, which dictate our genetic code. These extensions are called *dendrites* and *axons*. Axons are longer and allow communication with other more distant groups of neurons. These distances can be enormous. For example, the length of the axons your fingers require to turn these pages is probably about fifty inches.

Normally, the dendrites are numerous and serve as receivers of information from other neurons, either directly or via smaller neurons, termed interneurons, which extend numerous processes to nearby nerve cells. Such networking allows groups of neurons to be informed of the activity of nearby neighbors. Although neurons are the "business cells" of the brain, they are surrounded and outnumbered by a second class of cell, collectively termed *glia*. Glia do not

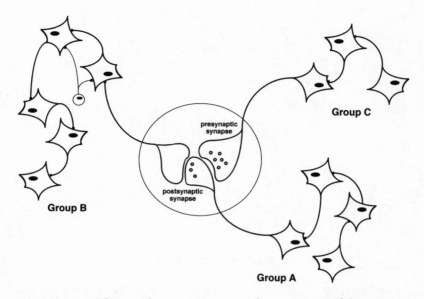

FIGURE 3.1. This simple cartoon envisions the interaction of three groups of brain neurons. The encircled area is an enlargement that shows the nature of their synaptic interactions. Group A interacts with group B using a postsynaptic synapse. Group C, by means of a presynaptic synapse, influences the extent of signaling between groups A and B. Each group has many interneurons that regulate the interactions of their component nerve cells. One such interneuron is represented by the small neuron shown in group B.

have the communicative ability of neurons but perform important functions in their maintenance.

The Greeks were convinced that the brain secreted fluids or "spirits" that flowed through the nerve axons to the muscles. Not until the late eighteenth century, when Luigi Galvani of Bologna had shown that frog muscles could be stimulated directly by electricity, was it considered that these "spirits" might be electrical signals. Later, in Germany, in 1850, Herman von Helmholtz determined the speed of the nerve electrical impulse to be about sixty miles per hour. Far too slow to be analogous to the mere physical passage of electricity through a wire, the nerve impulse had to be an active biological process.

In copper wires it is the movement of *electrons* within the copper atom that accounts for electrical currents. In contrast, electrical currents in biological systems are carried by *ions*, atoms that have become charged by the gain or loss of one or more electrons. But the number of ions inside a cell is not always the same as the number that exist outside the cell. For example, the concentration of sodium ions is higher outside the cell, and the concentration of potassium ions is highest inside. The membrane that surrounds the cell is polarized as a consequence of this unequal distribution of charged ions. The unequal distribution of ions creates two important physical forces. First, the differences in concentration generates a force that dictates the direction in which ions tend to move; they flow naturally from areas of higher concentration to areas where they are at a lower density. The second force depends on the natural tendency of ions to repel or attract one another. Ions with like charge, either positive or negative, repel each other; those with unlike charges are attracted together. *Electrostatic force* is the term used to refer to the affinity of ions for one another.

Furthermore, the differences in concentration of ions is believed to be due to the differing abilities of ions to pass freely through pores, or ion channels, in the cell membrane: some ions move unhindered, others with more difficulty. Their unequal distribution across the nerve cell membrane is maintained by some ions being ejected by the force of electrostatic repulsion and others by the action of small protein pumps in the membrane. The neuron therefore is like a tiny biological battery with the positive pole outside the cell and the negative pole inside—it maintains an electrical potential, a form of electrical pressure that can be measured in volts.

The electrical potential of a neuron is usually seventy millivolts; but if some event shifts this stasis, a sequence of reactions is triggered during which the nerve cell membrane briefly reverses its polarity. Sodium-selective channels in the cell membrane sense the voltage change and open suddenly, and this forces a rush of sodium ions into the neuron. The nerve cell becomes depolarized and is said to "fire." The sodium channels close quickly, in part aided by the opening of voltage-sensitive channels that are selective for potassium. The opening of these potassium channels allows the positively charged sodium ions to drive out the similarly charged potassium ions. Then, the normal unequal distribution of ions is restored, and the nerve cell becomes repolarized. This sequence of events generates a signal, termed an *action potential*, that is propagated along the entire length of the nerve cell through the sequential opening of sodium channels that sense the nearby voltage changes.

In terms of operation, a neuron is incredibly simple. It responds to many incoming electrical signals by sending out a stream of electrical impulses of its own. It is how this response changes with time and how it varies with the state of other parts of the brain that defines the unique complexity of our behavioral responses. The long-distance connections from one brain region to another are provided by large neurons, all of which are excitatory. The majority of these are referred to as *pyramidal cells* because of the triangular shape of their cell body. By virtue of their long axons, they can also inform and influence more distant regions to orchestrate other activities and generate an encompassing and unified response. By contrast, the interneurons are inhibitory and only exert local influence on neurons in the same neighborhood. Such networking allows groups of neurons to be informed of the activity of nearby neighbors. In this way, the community, or functional unit, can mount a coherent response.

Unfortunately, nerve cell dialogue is not always coherent. In some situations, such as epilepsy, certain neurons can start to fire in an erratic and uncontrolled manner. Epilepsy is usually the result of some damage to the nerve cells of a particular brain region, which can arise from concussion or damage from a toxic substance or infectious agent that has gained direct access to the brain. Axons arising from the area of excessive excitation also influence other, more distant groups of nerve cells, and eventually the whole brain can go into a state of uncontrolled nerve cell firing, which is termed a *seizure*. In this state the individual becomes incapacitated as a result of the loss of normal brain control over bodily functions, such as the ability to control the movement of muscles. These seizures are usually transient. Epilepsy was originally referred to as "lunacy" because it was believed to be influenced by the phases of the moon, but in some extreme cases seizures can occur continuously and become life threatening.

Fortunately, nowadays most conditions of epilepsy can be controlled using drugs designed specifically to alter the ion flow that is so crucial to nerve cell firing. The most powerful antiepilepsy drugs, such as phenytoin (Dilantin/Epanutin) or lamotrigine (Lamictal), prevent rapid closure of the sodium channels, and thus they slow down the recovery period and hence the frequency at which the nerve cell can fire. The converse is also true: the blockage of sodium channel opening inhibits nerve cell firing, with deadly consequences. For example, tetrodotoxin, which is found in the sex organs and gut of the puffer fish, the Japanese delicacy called *fugu*, specifically blocks the outer mouth of the sodium channel. A milligram or two of tetrodotoxin is lethal; smaller amounts numb sensation and weaken the limbs—an indication for believing that this is the active ingredient of the secret zombie death potion of voodoo rituals.

Mind the Gap

For many years it was believed that the electrical impulse passing down the axon simply jumped the gap between the nerve terminal and the adjacent nerve cell. While this remains true in certain cases,

evidence accumulating at the turn of the nineteenth century suggested that nerve cells were not in continuous contact but separated
by a specialized gap, which came to be termed the *synapse*. Around
the same time it was observed that simple chemical substances
could produce electrical excitability in cells. These combined observations led to the idea of *chemical neurotransmission*, a concept
finally accepted to be the most universal process of nerve cell
communication.

At the point where the axon terminates and makes the synapse,
the nerve ending expands into a more bulbous structure that contains many tiny sacks known as *vesicles*. This whole structure is
referred to as the *presynapse*. The vesicles contain chemicals that can
modify the excitability of the adjacent neuron, and because of this
action these chemicals are usually called *neurotransmitters*. The release of neurotransmitters is a specific and carefully controlled
process. The cell membrane of the presynapse is dotted with numerous calcium-selective ion channels that open only in response to the
voltage change. When these channels open, calcium ions enter the
presynapse and become involved in a mechanism that alters the surface of the vesicles. This allows the vesicles to fuse with the membrane of the nerve ending and spill their entire load of neurotransmitters into the synaptic gap.

As with tetrodotoxin, nature has evolved many exquisite systems
to effect this mechanism of transmission, enabling animals to
immobilize their prey. The marine cone snails from the Indo-Pacific
are renowned not only for the beauty of their shells but also for a
deadly toxin, known as *conotoxin*, which they inject into fish with a
hollow disposable tooth that serves as both harpoon and hypoder-
mic. This toxin blocks the mouth of the voltage-sensitive calcium
channel, preventing entry of calcium ions into the cell and the
release of neurotransmitters, with the concomitant loss of control
over neurotransmission. The unfortunate fish is rendered immobile
and eaten.

Once released, the neurotransmitters diffuse across the gap and interact with specific target sites, termed *receptors*, which are clustered on the adjacent, postsynaptic nerve cell at the point of contact with the presynapse. These receptors contain in their structure a specific docking site for a given neurotransmitter, much as a lock "recognizes" the proper key. This unique interaction, or binding, makes the synaptic process of chemical transmission very specific. A neurotransmitter cannot influence a cell that lacks receptors for it.

When a neurotransmitter is recognized by a receptor site, several things can happen, which depend largely on the nature of the receptor. Neurotransmitter and receptor interactions can trigger the opening or closing of an associated ion channel, which selectively allows the entry of one or more ions. For example, if sodium ions enter the *postsynaptic* nerve cell, it becomes electrically excited and generates an action potential. If chloride ions enter, firing is made more difficult because the inside of the cell becomes further polar-

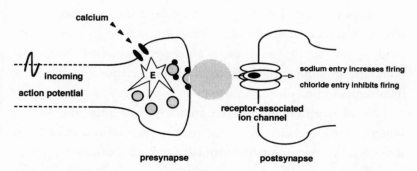

FIGURE 3.2. This diagram illustrates the basic features involved in the action of a neurotransmitter, such as glutamate or GABA, at a receptor that controls ion entry into a cell. When the axon potential arrives at the presynapse, calcium ions enter the cell and activate an enzyme (E). This modifies the vesicles in a manner that allows them to empty their transmitter load into the gap between the presynapse and the postsynaptic cell. The transmitter interacts with the receptor and opens the associated ion channel to allow the entry of either sodium or chloride ions into the postsynaptic cell.

ized by these negatively charged ions; it becomes harder to reverse the polarity and generate an action potential. In this state the nerve cell is said to become *hyperpolarized*. In many ways, these synaptic ion channels are quite similar to the ion-selective channels of the axon, but they differ significantly in that a chemical signal is needed to activate them rather than an electrical impulse.

Synaptic transmission is rapid and brief. As soon as the neurotransmitter interacts with its receptor, it is whisked away, clearing the field for the next burst of transmitter molecules to cross the synapse and initiate a new neuronal impulse. Neurotransmitters can be inactivated in the region of the synapse by enzymes. More frequently, neurotransmitters are pumped back into the axon that released them. This provides a unique conservation mechanism that allows these molecules to be used again and again. These mechanisms are crucial targets of drug action. Drugs used to treat depression prevent certain neurotransmitters from being pumped back into the presynapse; in this way, they enhance the action of the neurotransmitter by prolonging the period of time it remains within the synaptic gap. Other drugs, such as those used to treat schizophrenia, prevent the action of the neurotransmitter by blocking its binding site on the receptor. Such drugs are called *antagonists* because they inhibit the activation of the receptor and block its involvement in neurotransmission.

Not all receptors are located on the postsynaptic side of the synapse; some are located on the presynapse. Activation of these receptors, by incoming axon terminals from other neurons, can regulate the amount of neurotransmitters released (see figure 3.1). The pain-relieving action of morphine, for example, is derived from its ability to stimulate such receptors on the presynapse of neurons that conduct the sensation of pain. By activating these receptors, morphine lowers the amount of transmitter released and therefore reduces transmission of the pain signal. Because it mimicks the action of a naturally occurring neurotransmitter, morphine is said to be an *agonist*.

The brain contains many types of neurotransmitters. How they individually influence nerve firing so that our brain can generate an appropriate and coherent response to any given situation is the theme of the next chapter.

Neuronal Discourse

Currencies of the Mind

Since the action of neurotransmitters is to excite or inhibit nerve cell firing, it should not be too surprising that the relative excitability of nerve cells in the brain is dominated by two ubiquitous neurotransmitters. Both of these neurotransmitters are *amino acids*: *glutamate* causes nerve cell excitation, and *GABA* (gamma-aminobutyric acid) provides the opposite action of inhibition. These two neurotransmitters account for the action of the vast majority of nerve cells in the brain.

Brain glutamate is particularly interesting because this neurotransmitter can enhance communication between neighboring nerve cells when it is required that an excitatory response be enduring. Neurons have many receptors for glutamate, but two of them are of particular interest. These are termed the *AMPA* and *NMDA* receptors, the acronyms denoting the chemicals that research scientists use to activate preferentially the individual functions of each receptor. AMPA and NMDA receptors tend to coexist at many synapses, and they appear to act synergistically. Initially, transmitter glutamate acts only to effect the opening of the ion channel associated with the AMPA receptor. This allows entry, or gating, of sodium and potassium ions and results in the depolarization of the postsynaptic cell. Once depolarization has occurred, the NMDA receptor becomes responsive to the action of transmitter glutamate. In addition to sodium and potassium, however, its associated ion channel also allows calcium to enter the postsynaptic neuron. This is the determining step because the calcium sets in motion a whole cascade of molecular steps that stabilizes the enhanced synaptic response. Often this is referred to as a strengthening of the synapse, a phenomenon now known as *long-term potentiation* (LTP).

The majority of large neurons, the pyramidal cells, are excitatory and use glutamate as a neurotransmitter. The smaller interneurons are inhibitory and use GABA as a neurotransmitter. When GABA binds to its receptor, it produces fast inhibitory transmission by allowing the associated ion channel to gate chloride ions into the postsynaptic cell. This results in hyperpolarization and an inhibition of firing in the postsynaptic neuron. As a consequence, drugs that influence GABA receptor function can have profound effects on general excitability in the brain. Benzodiazepines, such as clonazepam, are useful in treating epilepsy because they counteract the excessive excitability by increasing the level of nerve cell inhibition. To achieve this effect, the benzodiazepines enhance the inhibitory effect of GABA at its receptor in a most remarkable way. They cause a change in the shape of the GABA receptor, which results in the GABA neurotransmitter binding with greater avidity. This has the effect of allowing more chloride ions to enter the cell, and the resultant increase in hyperpolarization makes further nerve cell firing more difficult. The converse is also true. Picrotoxin prevents the inhibitory actions of GABA. By blocking the mouth of the chloride channel regulated by the GABA receptor, inhibitory control is lost and severe convulsions ensue. These seizures can lead ultimately to death as they cause muscle spasms that restrict breathing and the appropriate contractions of the heart.

Thus the reciprocal actions of GABA and glutamate do most of the work to prevent nerve cells becoming totally silent or uncontrollably excited. This waxing and waning of excitability is easily recorded by placing electrical sensors at various points on the scalp to record the degree of excitability in the underlying cortex, that familiar rippled structure so often compared to a walnut. The readout comes in the form of waves that vary in their amplitude and frequency, which is measured in hertz (Hz), or oscillation per second. These so-called brain waves recorded as an electroencephalogram (EEG) are used to give an indication of the brain's activity, such as the degree of attention, wakefulness, or sleeping.

Mind and Body

But we need to explore how these states of arousal are governed—the mechanisms that dictate the degree of glutamate excitation or GABA inhibition. Given that the majority of brain neurons use one or the other of these neurotransmitters, some mechanism must exist to modulate their function. Otherwise it becomes difficult to account for the unique response of every individual in a given situation. These functional reactions are governed by clusters of nerve cells located in the lower regions of the brain where the spinal cord enters and expands in size to form the brain stem. Here exist groups of nerve cell bodies, the axons of which travel to all parts of the brain. Almost like vines, these axons envelop distant brain regions, their tendril-like endings curling around the component nerve cells. And these nerve terminals exert a profound modulatory influence on processes such as our sleep-waking cycles, movement, emotion, and learning.

In comparison with neurotransmission using glutamate and GABA, the general mode of chemical transmission employed by these nerve cells in the brain stem differs in two distinct ways. First, they use serotonin, noradrenaline, or dopamine as neurotransmitters. These chemical transmitters are constructed from amino acids, either tyrosine or tryptophan, by the action of enzymes specific to each nerve cell type. Second, the action of these transmitters at their receptors is different from that of either glutamate or GABA. When these transmitters bind to a receptor, there is no direct opening of an ion channel. Instead they modulate the activity of an enzyme on the inner postsynaptic face, and this leads to a cascade of events in the postsynaptic neuron. This cascade ultimately results in the opening of ion channels from the inside of the cell, change in cell polarity, and either excitation or inhibition of cell firing. As a consequence, this type of neurotransmission is much slower and more enduring. The nature of the receptor involved dictates whether the consequence of its activation will be excitation or inhibition. This is because some receptors cause activation of the associated enzyme and others cause its inhibition. These neurotransmitter systems have profound effects on the overall functioning of the brain.

The modulatory effects of these transmitter systems are exemplified nicely by considering the action of dopamine. Two groups of nerve cells in the brain stem use dopamine. One group, in an area

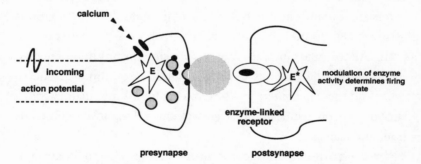

FIGURE 4.1. This diagram illustrates the basic features involved in the action of a neurotransmitter, such as serotonin or noradrenaline, at a receptor that regulates the opening of ion channels from the inside of the cell. When the neurotransmitter interacts with its receptor, it modulates the activity of an enzyme (E*) that in turn modulates ion entry into the postsynaptic cell and hence its state of polarisation.

called the *substantia nigra*, send their axons to brain regions involved in the control of movement. As mentioned above, these cells have degenerated in Parkinson's disease. The consequence of this condition is muscle tremor and rigidity due to an inability to initiate movement. Drugs can also have a significant effect on this dopamine system. The use of amphetamine results in hyperactivity and restlessness. This is because it slips into the vesicles of the presynapse and pushes out the dopamine transmitter in an uncontrolled manner. Extensive use of amphetamine, however, gives rise to a condition in which the user can become paranoid and delusional. These states are attributed to amphetamine releasing dopamine from axons arising from the second group of neurons that use dopamine, in the region of the brain stem called the *ventral tegmental area*. These dopamine-containing axons influence brain regions associated with how we evaluate the information in our surroundings, and excessive activity can result in irrational thought processes. Dopamine malfunctions in this region of the brain occur in schizophrenia, a topic to which we shall return later.

By contrast, the actions of serotonin and noradrenaline are much more involved in brain-mind activation. Noradrenaline enlivens our state of vigilance; it enhances our response and attention to the surrounding stimuli in our environment. Noradrenaline-containing axons arise from a small group of neurons, containing about 10,000 cells, which extend to influence many brain regions. This group of neurons is located in a region of the brain stem called the *locus coeruleus*, and, as the name implies, it is an exquisite colour of blue. Nearby, another group of neurons, termed the *raphe nucleus*, use serotonin to modulate distant areas of the brain. Both serotonin and noradrenaline seem to regulate our mood. Many antidepressant drugs, such as Prozac (fluoxetine), seem to improve mood because they enhance the action of these transmitters. These drugs block neurotransmitter inactivation by preventing their reuptake into the presynapse.

Serotonin and noradrenaline also regulate sleep and dreaming. During sleep the oscillations on the EEG are slow. But in some alternating periods, known as rapid-eye-movement (REM) sleep, the EEG oscillations look more awake than asleep as they occur more quickly. This is the dreaming phase of sleep—and serotonin and noradrenaline regulate its duration. Serotonin has also been linked to aggression. The activity of this neurotransmitter seems to be unusually low in individuals who have taken, or have attempted to take, their own lives by violent means such as firearms or jumping from heights, as compared with those who have ingested poison or a drug overdose. Serotonin and noradrenaline exert complex effects, and we are only beginning to understand the magnitude of their influence on the brain.

There is, however, one other aspect of brain function that is so obvious it is seldom mentioned: the brain is attached to the body. When nerve cells outside the brain detect decreasing levels of sugar in the bloodstream, they send a signal to the brain that initiates the behavioral response of eating. The connection also works the other way. Mental states can have a profound effect on the body. For example, individuals with phobias frequently experience sweating of the palms.

Brain activity gives rise to chemical signals, which can alter the function of many cells and tissues, as well as the regulatory circuits that initiated the cycle itself. Our emotional response to fear, for example, is dependent on a brain structure called the *amygdala*. The amygdala, along with the hippocampus, snuggle under the lateral temporal lobes of the cortex. Activation of the amygdala quickens the firing of neurons, whose axons extend from the brain into the body, where they trigger the release of adrenaline from glands located near each kidney. The released adrenaline influences many bodily functions, such as heart rate and muscle tone, but it also arouses brain function by activating nerve cells that reenter the brain stem and stimulate the noradrenaline-containing neurons of the locus coeruleus.

The ever-changing flow of brain and bodily chemicals dictates our sense of awareness, mood, and emotion. It is not unreasonable to believe that drugs contribute further to the complex mechanisms of our minds.

5

Nostri Plena Laboris

The Emotional Past

We do not know when humans started using caffeine or nicotine. Tea, coffee, cola, and cocoa are but some beverages consumed for their stimulating actions. All derive their effects from caffeine and, to a lesser extent, theophylline and theobromine, which are related to caffeine in both structure and action. Similarly, nicotine has been extracted by chewing, smoking, or snorting an array of plant leaves or seeds to obtain its stimulant actions. All have been employed in most cultures since antiquity.

Tea drinking probably originated in China at the time of the Yellow Emperor, the Divine Healer, some 5,000 years ago, but the first authenticated use in the West was about 1,600 years ago. Coffee originated in Ethiopia and was brought to Saudi Arabia and domesticated around 1,400 years ago, as was extensively documented by Avicenna, a Persian philosopher in the eleventh century. In South America *erva mate* was brewed by the Guarani Indians of Brazil for hundreds of years, using extracts from the leaves of *Ilex paraguayensis*. Of equal antiquity is the potent guarana drink prepared in the Amazon region from the seeds of a woody liana known as *Paullinia cuprana*. The tree from which cocoa is derived, originally native to the Amazon valley but brought to Mexico in pre-Hispanic times, provided the Aztecs with *chocolatl,* their famed "food of the gods."

The story of nicotine and related stimulants is similar. The habit of betel-nut chewing has been around continuously in areas spanning east Africa to Polynesia, and later into India. The term *betel nut* is a misnomer. The substance chewed actually consists of seeds from the palm *Areca catechu* wrapped in the leaves of the vine *Piper betel* along with some lime juice to aid the release of arecaidine, the active component, which has nicotine-like actions. Chewing the betel nut produces copious quantities of red substance, which stains the teeth. Such stained teeth have been seen in a skeleton estimated to be about 5,000 years old.

Chewing khat leaves (*Catha edulis*) for the stimulatory properties of its active ingredient, cathinone, has its origins in Ethiopia, and the habit extended to Somalia and the Yemen, where it remains to this day. Pituri, a nicotine-containing extract from the *Duboisia hopwoodii* shrub, whether chewed or smoked, has been prized for centuries by the Australian aborigines. However, "white fella pituri" is principally an American phenomenon, the cultural use of which dates back to the prehistory of South America. It probably emerged there some 5,000 to 7,000 years ago and spread as far north as Alaska, where the Tlingit were found to be chewing tobacco when they first came in contact with Europeans. This small group of Native Americans, culturally defined by the use of a distinct language, lived in an environment with easy access to an abundance of food. Their use of tobacco was not to stave off hunger—it must have served more social functions.

Amphetamine is more modern in origin. It was developed for the relief of asthma because of its ability to dilate the airways and passages of the lungs. Originally, adrenaline was used, but the need to inject it prompted the Lilly drug company to investigate an old Chinese herbal remedy for asthma, *ma huang* (*Ephedra vulgaris*). Its researchers isolated ephedrine from this remedy, and it was found to aid in the relief of asthma when taken orally. A purely synthetic substitute was required, as *ma huang* was a scarce commodity. Gordon Alles, in the mid-1930s, came up with the answer in the form of amphetamine, which was marketed as Benzedrine. The amphetamine synthesized by Alles contained two chemicals that were mirror images of each other. One, called dexamphetamine, was much more potent and was eventually marketed as Dexedrine. Because amphetamine could be prepared in a volatile form, the Benzedrine inhaler was developed for asthmatics by Smith, Kline and French and sold widely as a nonprescription drug in the 1930s and 1940s. Of course, the inhaler was broken open and the contents swallowed for their stimulant effects.

But chewing the contents of Benzedrine inhalers was not the cause of the major epidemic of amphetamine abuse that followed. During World War II amphetamines were frequently administered to keep pilots awake during night air raids and given to civilians to boost their productivity in wartime industries. Even Hitler is reported to have had an amphetamine abuse problem—this may have contributed to his psychotic-like madness. In the years following the end of World War II, amphetamine use was so common that it was featured in songs of the time, such as "Who Put Benzedrine in Mrs. Murphy's Ovaltine?" The popularity of amphetamines reached an apogee in the hippie era of the late 1960s with the so-called amphetamine runs—injections every two hours for three to six days. In the United States alone, the legal production of amphetamine exceeded ten billion tablets in the early 1970s.

Stimulating Legacies

Amphetamine-type stimulants still remain popular, but their fashion tends to be one of abuse. New forms continue to emerge from underground laboratories with alarming rapidity, owing to the relative ease of synthesis, freely available starting chemicals, and recipes accessible on the Internet. The number of current users of amphetamine-like substances is estimated to be about 0.5 percent of the global population. In comparison with the 1970s amphetamine era, perhaps we should simply consider continuing uses of amphetamine-like substances to be a contained but enduring fashion.

Their use is increasing, however. One form of amphetamine that has gained recent notoriety is methylenedioxymethamphetamine, popularly known as ecstasy. It is central to an amazing rave-scene subculture where users dance the night away and drink vast quantities of soft drinks to stave off dehydration. The mood-altering qualities of ecstasy appear to be dependent on its ability specifically to release serotonin, the mood molecule of the brain, from nerve endings. Originally, serotonin was believed to control bodily function because it was identified by its ability to regulate contractions of muscle and intestine and to control blood pressure by constricting blood vessels. Later, in the 1950s, drugs that reduced serotonin levels were found to depress the mood of patients, and this is the main reason for concern about ecstasy. When taken regularly, ecstasy may cause irreversible damage to nerve cells that use serotonin. As the raphe nucleus of the brain stem incorporates 165,000 serotonin-containing nerve cells, a tiny fraction of the billions of nerve cells that make up the brain, the long-term consequences of prolonged ecstasy use are likely to be altered states of mood in later life.

Methylphenidate (Ritalin) is another amphetamine-related drug that is currently used for the treatment of so-called attention-deficit hyperactivity disorder (ADHD) in children. It may seem paradoxical that methylphenidate, a stimulant, can be used to treat hyperactivity, but the prevailing view is that the calming effects of the drug arise from its ability to increase serotonin levels and so improve mood. Another current fad is the use of amphetamine-like compounds for weight loss. Amphetamines, on average, can reduce initial body weight by about 10 percent. Drugs such as dexfenflu-

ramine (Redux), fenfluramine (Pondimin), and phentermine (Ion-
amin) are thought to exert their slimming, or anorexic, effects by
increasing the release of serotonin. Some neurotransmitters tell
us when our stomachs are full, serotonin makes us feel satisfied.
The popularity of drug combinations containing fenfluramine
and phentermine, popularly known as "fen/phen," however, was ill
fated: reports of drugs causing blood to leak through heart valves
resulted in their withdrawal from the market.

By contrast, the consumption of milder stimulants, such as caffeine, nicotine, and related substances is embedded in our culture
and is of far greater social significance. The folklore surrounding
their use is very often associated with the meditations of holy men,
who also valued them for their medicinal properties. But gradually
they took on a social importance.

In the fifteenth century the tea ceremony became an integral
part of the Zen Buddhist culture of the Japanese, who adopted
many Chinese customs. During the social rites of the Aborigines,
known as "big talks," *pituri* is chewed and passed from mouth to
mouth in order of community status. Khat houses tend to attract
specific customers—for example, some for truck drivers, others for
civil servants. And the use of stimulants has led to the development
of finely crafted instruments. The legendary calumets, or "peace
pipes," of the Native Americans used on important social and ceremonial occasions were adorned with all sorts of symbolic features,
including feathers and locks of women's hair. Another example of
artisan craft associated with the use of stimulants is the betel cutter.
This hinged, one-bladed instrument was designed solely to cut the
arecaidine-containing "nut." All knives have a similar function, but
their design and decoration can be seen as a sort of microcosm of
Asian metalwork, with the craftspeople of a dozen different cultures
producing items that are similar in function and general shape but
utterly different in design and workmanship. Betel has been the
inspiration for these minor art forms in Asia.

So why did Europe not embrace tea, coffee, and nicotine as social stimulants until the fifteenth century? Their use could not have spread naturally to Europe since the land-bridge between Siberia and Alaska was lost when the ice sheets retreated some 12,000 years ago, well in advance of documented use of stimulants in the Americas. But Europe's enduring preoccupation with alcohol may have been the most important contributing factor. While winemaking may have had its origins in the Middle East, the Romans made Europe its home, and the Church remained the repository of these Roman skills during the Dark Ages. The use of alcohol was actively pursued in Europe over the centuries in a hedonistic manner, in the Saxon ale taverns, the absinthe shops of Southern France, and the gin houses of London. Other than alcohol, there appears to be no record of drug use in Western Europe, except for the lethal and sickening plant extracts of black henbane, mandrake, and deadly nightshade, to which have been attributed the frenzied flights of witches. And in Northern Europe and Asia the use of the fly agaric mushroom (*Amanita muscaria*) for its inebriant properties proliferated. The introduction of caffeine and nicotine to Europe had to await recovery from the collapse of the ancient world and the beginnings of a huge expansion of trading.

The Tang dynasty extended its control far into Central Asia, and emergent Islam stretched its empire from the shores of the Atlantic to Afghanistan and beyond. The Silk Road connected the Mediterranean with China; and the Muslims developed sea routes from the Red Sea to India and Indonesia and overland routes across the Sahara to the kingdoms of Black Africa. In Europe, toward the end of the fifteenth century, the voyages of Vasco da Gama, Magellan, and Columbus opened up sea routes to the Far East and the Americas. They developed the necessary nautical skills that enabled European ships to transport silver from the Americas, porcelain from China, and spices from the East Indies to the flourishing cities of western Europe. The Iberian colonialism and imperialism of the eighteenth and nineteenth centuries followed the 1494 agreement, established under the auspices of the Pope, that divided the world for the purposes of exploration and settlement. Access to lands east of a longitude in the Atlantic was to be restricted to Portugal, and areas west of the line belonged to Spain. By the end of the sixteenth century, the English and Dutch followed the Portuguese route around Southern Africa and on to India and Persia. Moreover, they ferried commodities, obtained by the Spanish in Central America, from Seville to Amsterdam and London for further use in their trade with the Far East.

One cannot overstate the historical significance of the introduction to Europe of stimulants such as coffee, tea, chocolate, and nicotine brought by the enterprising merchants of the seventeenth century. Coffee houses and cafés opened up by the thousands. Parisian café society became firmly rooted. Alcohol consumption was reduced and industriousness enhanced. In short, the use of stimulants achieved chemically what rationalism and the Protestant ethic sought to fulfil spiritually and ideologically (though some religious leaders such as John Wesley originally decried that tea was a "drug"). So the deployment of caffeine meshed perfectly with the ideals and values of the Enlightened society. Trade escalated to supply the increasing demands. The cultivation of coffee spread rapidly beyond the confines of Northeast Africa and Arabia into other suitable areas with hot climates and heavy rainfall. The Dutch planted coffee in Java and Ceylon at the end of the seventeenth century, and seeds from a single tree maintained in a botanical garden in Amsterdam served the plantations in Surinam and French Guiana and the establishment of the enormous Brazilian coffee industry in the early eighteenth century.

The introduction of tea was somewhat different. The Dutch introduced it to France and Germany in the early seventeenth century, where it was fashionable for only a brief period; tea still does not appear to be popular in wine-growing countries. But the British embraced it after its first public sale in 1657. This popularity led both to large-scale smuggling and to adulteration, or "smouching," of tea with hedge clippings and other plant detritus. In 1826 "Honest" John Horniman and other tea merchants standardized the quality of tea by selling it in sealed packets of guaranteed weight and purity. Tea grew popular in North America through trade with the Netherlands, and in Russia through trade with China. But this trade had its difficulties. The British developed tea cultivation in India as a way of breaking the Chinese monopoly, and the first sale of Assam tea occurred in London in 1839. Since the powerful British East India Company was prevented from reexporting tea from Britain to America, it forced the passing of the Regulating Act of 1773, which withdrew the export duty on tea. This offended powerful interests in the American colonies. British ships were raided and their cargo dumped into the sea at the so-called Boston Tea Party, one of the events that triggered the American War of Independence.

Jean Nicot de Villemain is generally credited, although probably undeservedly, with bringing tobacco to Europe in 1560, and he fought to have the plant (*Nicotiana tabacum*) named after him. The use of tobacco was adopted enthusiastically and, by the beginning of the seventeenth century, it was no longer an exotic custom but an integral part of social life. James Rolfe initiated its cultivation in Virginia in 1612, and the exports required to supply the thousands of retail outlets soared from 9 tons in 1617 to 230 tons in 1627. Initially, pipe smoking was popular, but snorting finely ground tobacco, known as "snuff," soon superseded this. Snuff was purchased according to grain size and fragrance, imparted by the use of various additives. Cigars, the original form of tobacco smoking, were developed mainly by the Dutch in Southeast Asia, and their use spread from Holland throughout Europe around 1830, owing largely to favorable taxation. Chewing tobacco, the original method of use, was not adopted widely and remained an American habit. Another European invention was the cigarette. Developed in Spain and Portugal, the use of cigarettes increased dramatically during World War I and II when they were supplied in large quantities to troops, no doubt for their stimulant qualities, which helped to stave off hunger and fatigue.

The beneficial qualities of tobacco have been hotly debated for centuries and, probably, long before it was introduced to Western society. King James I of England wrote "A Counterblaste to Tobacco" and published it anonymously in 1604. He condemned tobacco as "A custom loathsome to the eye, hateful to the nose, harmful to the braine, dangerous to the lungs, and in the black stinking fumes thereof, nearest resembling the horrible Stygian smoke of the pit that is bottomless." He chastised users by imposing a fortyfold tax increase on the purchase of tobacco. This penalty failed to dissuade many from promoting the benefits of smoking tobacco. In 1659 Dr. Giles Everard wrote: "To strengthen the memory the smoke is excellent taken by the nostrils, for it is properly belonging to the brain, and it is easily conveyed into the cells of it and it cleanseth that from all filth (for the brain is the Metropolis of phlegm, as Hippocrates teacheth us)." Despite epidemiological evidence since the 1950s of ill health associated with the use of cigarettes, attempts to curb tobacco use are still minimal. Tobacco remains a popular stimulant. To quote Oscar Wilde: "A cigarette is the perfect type of a perfect pleasure. It is exquisite and it leaves one unsatisfied."

Memory Mediators

Caffeine

Caffeine is a remarkable substance. It is present in tea, coffee, and cola, drinks that form an integral part of our daily routine. An average cup of coffee contains about eighty milligrams of pure caffeine, and tea contains about half that amount. Most people are aware of the arousing effects of caffeine: it increases our blood pressure and heart rate, improves our concentration and flow of thought, and wards off sleep. It provides a regular way to start the day. And its use continues throughout the day in all forms of social interaction, from business meetings to the welcoming of both friends and strangers. Our daily consumption of pure caffeine is often more than half a gram. All of it will have been completely absorbed into the bloodstream, where it will remain for between two and five hours following each cup of coffee or tea.

The effects of caffeine on the brain are even more remarkable. It antagonizes the action of a substance known as *adenosine*, which broadly depresses nerve cell activity. Adenosine slows our motor activity, depresses respiration, and induces sleep, all of which are precise opposites of the effects of caffeine. Adenosine is an unusual regulator of brain function. It is probably not a neurotransmitter because it has no defined synthetic pathway and is not stored in synaptic vesicles. It is more a chemical mediator that modulates general brain function.

The main source of adenosine is from the breakdown of *ATP* (adenosine triphosphate), which is the general source of energy in the body. It can be produced from both inside and outside the nerve cells and glia. This makes the identification of the brain pathways that use adenosine a daunting task: the inhibitory actions of adenosine on nerve-cell firing extend throughout the brain, where it inhibits the release of many neurotransmitters, including noradrenaline, dopamine, GABA, and glutamate. It also inhibits the release of other chemical mediators, such as adrenaline. In essence, adenosine dampens neuronal excitability, thereby reducing our state of brain and bodily arousal.

In the brain adenosine acts on at least three receptors, the A1, A2, and A3 receptors. Caffeine is an effective antagonist at the A1 and A2 receptors, but not at the A3 receptor, the function of which is little understood. Antagonism of the A2 receptor explains the restlessness produced by caffeine because this receptor is found mainly in the striatum, a brain region intimately involved in the regulation of movement. By contrast, antagonism of the A1 receptor is believed to account for the arousing effects of caffeine because these receptors are densely distributed in the cortex and, notably, in the hippocampus, a structure that plays an important role in learning. Here caffeine blocks the inhibitory action of adenosine at concentrations achieved with one or two cups of coffee. Excitatory neurotransmission is increased by the enhanced release of glutamate. In experimental models adenosine facilitates the occurence of LTP, a model for the molecular mechanisms of memory.

Caffeine is generally thought to improve the speed of our reactions and the ability to perform simple calculations or the learning of strings of syllables. However, some researchers dispute these findings. They argue that the individuals serving as the control group would have been caffeine free, and withdrawal from the drug would have hindered their performance. This is an interesting view because it suggests that we all are caffeine dependent.

Nicotine

Nicotine is another commonly used drug that has arousing effects not unlike those of caffeine. About ten minutes after a cigarette, nicotine levels are at their maximum. Heart rate and blood pressure increase, and adrenaline is released. The brain waves, or EEG, of the cortex quickly assume an alerted pattern that indicates a state of arousal. The uptake of blood glucose into the brain is enhanced, leading to increased metabolic activity and energy use. Fatigue is reduced and cognitive performance enhanced. Simple motor-skill tasks are improved. But the effects of nicotine on problem-solving tasks are unclear—some researchers report an improvement, and others report no effect.

Nicotine can affect molecular processes of memory that are

modulated by an *acetylcholine* neurotransmitter system. Unlike the axons of the serotonin, dopamine, and noradrenaline systems that ascend from the brain stem, those employing acetylcholine arise from a group of neurons in the basal forebrain—the so-called nucleus basalis of Meynert—and extend to influence brain regions, such as the hippocampus and cortex, which are involved in learning and memory. Acetylcholine can act on two receptor types. Receptors of the so-called muscarinic type mediate slow neurotransmission, whereas those activated by nicotine, the nicotinic receptors, mediate fast neurotransmission. There are many varieties of nicotinic acetylcholine receptors, and those located on the presynapse have a unique structure that permits the entry of calcium ions. Since these receptors are located on neurons that release glutamate, their stimulation results in increased levels of glutamate, the activation of the NMDA receptors, and increased excitation. A single cigarette can achieve this excitation, which may account for some of the arousing effects it induces. The nicotinic receptors have another unusual feature: they very quickly become unresponsive, or desensitized, to the effects of nicotine and enter a long-lasting inactive state. This may explain the discrepancies observed with nicotine in problem-solving tasks, and it is probably the reason why the first cigarette of the day is renowned to be the best—the receptors have just "recovered" from the previous day's onslaught.

Cocaine and Amphetamine

Robert Louis Stevenson wrote his fascinating tale *The Strange Case of Dr. Jekyll and Mr. Hyde* in six days and nights. Rumor has it that he was using cocaine. Sigmund Freud, another cocaine user, believed it "steels one to intellectual effort." How much did cocaine contribute to the development of his psychoanalytic theories?

High doses of amphetamine have similar effects. Amphetamine, at a dose of seventy to eighty milligrams, increases alertness, confidence, and concentration and produces a general sense of well being. But doubling the dose often leads to a state of unease or mental discomfort, sometimes referred to as *dysphoria*, accompanied by social withdrawal and depression. If such high doses are continued, individuals begin to engage in repetitious thoughts or meaningless acts for hours on end and are often preoccupied with their own thought processes or some grand philosophical concern. They can become suspicious, antisocial, and even violent. Repetitive movements occur, such as continuous chewing or grinding of teeth. Psychotic reactions can develop. Typically, these consist of visual and auditory experiences or paranoia accompanied by delusions of persecution. In severe cases the user may perceive parasites under the skin and will frantically pick and gouge at it to remove the imagined pest. Was the demonic, murdering Mr. Hyde partly modelled on a cocaine user? Clearly, these drugs are powerful stimulants and not for the faint hearted.

In the brain amphetamine works by increasing noradrenaline and, particularly, dopamine activity. This is achieved in two different ways. First, amphetamine can diffuse into the nerve endings and "push" the neurotransmitters from their storage sites in the synaptic vesicles because its chemical structure closely resembles that of the neurotransmitters. Second, while it is not sufficiently similar to either dopamine or noradrenaline to activate their receptors, it can cause the activation of these neurotransmitters by blocking the pump that normally sequesters them back into the presynapse for subsequent reuse. The overall effect of cocaine is the same, but it seems to act specifically by blocking the reuptake pump rather than displacing transmitters from their storage sites. Enhanced noradrenaline activity has an alerting effect in the cortex and hippocampus, whereas increased dopamine levels may account for some of the other effects of cocaine and amphetamine, in particular movement disorders and psychosis. The difference between cocaine and amphetamine is that the latter has a more enduring effect.

TABLE 5.I Neurotransmitter Systems Influenced by Psychostimulant Drugs

Agent	Transmitter(s) affected
Miscellaneous stimulants	
Caffeine Theophylline Theobromine	Adenosine antagonists
Nicotine	Acetylcholine agonist
Arecaidine	Inhibits GABA reuptake?
Amphetamine-type stimulants	
Ephedrine Amphetamine Dexamphetamine Cocaine Methylphenidate Cathinone	Increase noradrenaline and dopamine release
Methylenedioxyamphetamine Fenfluramine Dexfenfluramine Phentermine	Increase serotonin release

So how do these different drug-taking behaviors program our brain? There is no simple answer to this question. We all have an inherent capacity to learn from experience; our genes provide us with this ability. But the power to record our experiences in the brain must depend on some particular properties of nerve cells that allow us to adapt to the social circumstances of life. The consumption of stimulant-containing beverages, for example, is a learned behavior. These beverages contain bitter tannins, which do not make them attractive drinks for children; the taste for tea and coffee is acquired slowly. Initially, the social use of stimulants is observed by children.

However, as sexual maturity advances, the need to become involved in adult discussion and to assert their views results invariably in experimentation with and assimilation of the pleasing warmth and stimulant qualities of beverages like tea and coffee. This new behavior allows adolescents to acquire the necessary etiquette of conversation, sociability, and communicative skills. The process of learning etiquette could be considered an adaptive phenomenon that generates kinship and serves possibly to identify and attract future partners. In other words, it enhances the individual's potential for survival. It is not always obvious why behavioral traits, such as drinking tea and coffee, are retained. Yet this behavioral trait seems to have been faithfully transmitted. It may be that humans have used bitter plant extracts since prehistory for the sole purpose of stimulating communication. It may also be possible that caffeine has altered our prior experiences since it competes with neurotransmitters to modify neural activity.

Great artifacts and images have transcended the basic simplicity of stimulant use. Stimulants are associated with crafted artifacts, ranging from finely carved meerschaum pipes to ornate French snuffboxes made of gold, and from the German porcelain of Meissen to the samovars of Russia. They contribute to our images of "men of steel"—Churchill with a Havana cigar or Stalin with his English briar pipe—or of heroes and heroines: the sultry cigarettes of Lauren Bacall and Humphrey Bogart reinforce behaviors that advocate stimulant use. It would seem that the use of stimulants has become firmly embedded in the conscious realm of our minds, intricately interwoven in a manner that, over time, has become a significant part of our culture. One could be forgiven for considering our propensity for stimulant use an inherited trait.

6

An Abyss Yawns

Valuta

If you want to know the abuse potential of any drug, check out its "street" value. As a simple example, the price of a quarter of a kilogram of tea is, on average, half that of the same weight of coffee. This price difference may relate partly to their manufacture and distribution, but it mainly reflects their caffeine content. Opium provides an even more fascinating example. Addiction was only one of the problems to which opium gave rise in nineteenth-century China—wars were fought over it and an imperial dynasty trembled as China's social and cultural structure was threatened.

Consider the following. Emperor Tsung Chen prohibited tobacco smoking in the mid–seventeenth century, so the Chinese population turned to opium. When supplies ran low, the insatiable demand was met by Warren Hastings, the British Governor General of Bengal in the 1770s. Trade grew brisk. The British East India Company, along with American merchants, continued to satisfy the need by smuggling opium into China through the port of Canton, at about 1,000,000 pounds sterling per annum. The late Ch'ing Dynasty government was in power in China, and there was grave social and economic disruption because of the ever-spreading opium habit. The emperor Tao-Kuang appointed a radical patriot,

Lin Tse-Hsu, as Imperial Commissioner of an antiopium campaign. When he arrived in Canton in March 1839, Lin destroyed more than 20,000 chests of opium. Fighting ensued—huge profits were at stake. In February 1840 the British Governor decided to send an expedition under Rear Admiral George Elliot to sort out the mess. The Chinese did not stand a chance against the Royal Navy—they had no concept of modern warfare and were undertrained and underequipped. The Treaty of Nanking was signed on August 29, 1842, and the Treaty of Bogue on October 8, 1843; an enormous indemnity was paid, and China was required to close five trading ports.

Around 1906, when an estimated 13.5 million Chinese smoked opium, questions about the morality of the trade arose, and Britain resolved to reduce exports of Indian opium to China. However, it was the introduction of opium into North and South America and Australia by Chinese immigrants that finally persuaded the various governments that action to curb its use had to be taken. The International Opium Commission was inaugurated in 1909, and by 1914 thirty-four nations had agreed to curb opium production and importation. World War I then intervened, and at the next meeting of the Commission in 1924, the number of countries that had agreed to some form of control had risen to sixty-two. In the end the newly formed League of Nations took over the task of controlling opium and, among other resolutions, declared that all signatory countries should pass effective laws or regulations to limit its use exclusively for medical and scientific purposes. Admirable goals, but they were of little consequence to the poor farmers in the so-called Golden Crescent (Afghanistan, Iran, Pakistan) and Golden Triangle (Laos, Myanmar [formerly Burma], and Thailand)—for them the unlawful production of opium was more worthwhile than subsistence farming. The illicit trade continues to flourish today. World opium production more than doubled in the ten-year period between 1982 and 1992. More than 160 years have passed since

Lin Tse-Hsu's aggressive campaign, but there is still no abatement in the opium trade. It continues to expand rapidly to supply a seemingly insatiable demand.

The Veiled Trade

For the unlawful drug trade to flourish, it needs to adapt continually to change in the world's political economy and advances in technology. In recent years Afghanistan and Myanmar have dominated the cultivation of the opium poppy (*Papaver somniferum*) and account for roughly three-quarters of global opium production. The unripened poppy-seed head is lanced and the resulting milky juice, termed *opium* from the Greek word for juice, is collected on several successive days. The sticky mess contains up to 20 percent by weight of a plant chemical known as *morphine*. About one-third of the juice is used as opium, and the rest is retained for the extraction of morphine and its conversion into heroin in clandestine laboratories. In the past these were located primarily in Europe, near the source of the necessary chemicals. Today the production process takes place close to the poppy fields, where the risks of detection are perceived to be lower. Here morphine is extracted using lime and ammonia and converted into heroin when acetic acid is bonded to the morphine. Following the removal of impurities with water and chloroform, the final and most difficult stage is the conversion of heroin into powder form. This requires considerable technical skill because the process requires the use of ether, which is explosive.

Trafficking is the crucial link in the chain between drug production and consumption, and it incurs the highest proportion of costs associated with the industry. In general, groups operating in Southwest Asia supply the bulk of the European heroin market, while those operating in Southeast Asia supply the market in North America. The associated "transaction costs" can easily rise to more than 90 percent of the market retail price. At this level the illicit

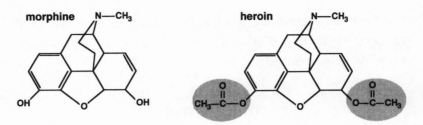

FIGURE 6.1. The structure of morphine and heroin is quite similar except for the modification (shaded areas) produced by the action of acetic acid.

drug economy and organized crime become more or less interdependent. Organizations, such as the Sicilian Mafia and the Colombian Medellin cartel, provide and invest the necessary capital and use violence as a management tool. But "narco-dollar" laundering is the most pervasive aspect of the unlawful drug trade. Until the retail proceeds are "purified" of their traces, they represent a major liability to the trafficker or dealer.

The process of money laundering requires the penetration of economic, political, and administrative sectors, and this can have a detrimental impact on activities that would normally promote rapid growth in trade and economic development. The requirement for financial centers to complete a Suspicious Transaction Report, an international agreement for large-scale cash dealings, is circumvented by the practice of "smurfing" by which smaller tranches of money are invested without the need for justification. The use of "front," or "shell," companies is another mechanism. Front companies are usually cash intensive, such as restaurants, bars, and nightclubs, which facilitates over- or underinvoicing. Shell companies enable the deposit of funds in offshore accounts from which they may be repatriated to repay a legitimate bank loan. Moreover, the drugs traded form their own currency, and are provided by or discounted in payment for services ranging from prostitution to protection and all varieties of criminal acts. Paying for these disruptive activities with a substance that itself engenders more illicit behaviour exacts an even higher toll on the community.

Into the Arms of Morpheus

As recently as the mid-1970s, a rationale for the compulsive use of morphine began to evolve. Initially, Solomon Snyder and Candace Pert at Johns Hopkins University, in Baltimore, demonstrated that morphine acts on defined receptors in the brain in a very specific way. We now know that there are at least three distinct receptors—termed the *mu, kappa*, and *delta* receptors—and that morphine acts to varying extents on all three, the *mu* receptor being the preferred one. These are generally referred to as the *opiate receptors*, because morphine, heroin, and their related modern counterparts—the opiates or opioids—exert their action at these receptors.

Almost in parallel, an explanation for the existence of these receptors was established by John Hughes and Hans Kosterlitz at the University of Aberdeen, in Scotland. This was the discovery of a family of unique neurotransmitters called the enkephalins, endorphins, and dynorphins, now referred to collectively as *endorphins*. Each endorphin is composed of a string of amino acids, or peptides, obtained from a relatively large protein precursor, which is split into the active peptides by enzymes. While their physiological role is not fully understood, they are believed to make up a highly specialized chemical signaling system that acts upon the opiate receptors under particular environmental circumstances. This neurotransmitter system is located particularly in regions that modulate pain perception and respiration, mainly the spinal cord and brain stem, but it is also part of areas that control our emotional state, such as the amygdala. In contrast to morphine, these peptides prefer the *delta* receptors and tend not to produce the resultant drug-seeking behavior. This makes morphine a rather special exception because its preferred action on the *mu* receptors can lead to the addicted state.

This opiate signaling system has become synonymous with the "fight or flight" concept, mainly because of its unsurpassed ability to block the perception of pain, an effect called *analgesia*. The most obvious protective function of this system is in situations where pain may block escape from a damage-inducing source. The pain transmitted from receptors located on the skin, or close to the surface of the body, is usually intense but involves little emotional reaction. On the other hand, pain that is deeper, arising from the body's organs, is poorly localized, pervasive, and has a strong emotional content. As such, it can signal, or presage, a pathological condition. A patient receiving morphine will maintain that such pain is as intense as ever but no longer offensive. The ability of morphine to modify the emotional component of pain probably explains why it is more effective in alleviating chronic, or pathological, pain than brief episodes of acute pain.

The dual nature of pain, that combination of sensory and emotional components, is reflected by the pain-relieving action of morphine in separate brain pathways. Acute pain sensed by the body's pain receptors increases the firing of their nerve cells, and transmission of this signal is blocked by morphine at the point where the nerve cells enter the spinal cord. If the action is presynaptic, it arises from a decrease in the entry of calcium ions through the voltage-sensitive ion channels and failure to release the neurotransmitter; if postsynaptic, it enhances potassium ion outflow, and the cell becomes hyperpolarized and cannot fire. However, nerve cell axons descending from the raphe nucleus in the brain stem can also modulate pain perception. Likewise, the axons of the pain pathway that enter the brain from the spinal cord influence the perception of pain and may be responsible for its emotional content. The action of morphine in these higher control centers therefore can reduce the emotional content of pain.

The existence of myriad interconnecting pain pathways explains why there is no simple relationship between analgesia and opioid action. This has been highlighted by research into the mechanisms of acupuncture, the ancient Chinese method for relief of pain. The technique involves the rhythmic movement of metallic needles inserted into the skin to reach deep structures such as muscles and tendons. Although it can facilitate endorphin release—an action that can be blocked by naloxone, an opiate antagonist—this is not a general phenomenon but depends on the characteristics of the acupuncture procedure employed. Furthermore, psychosocial factors are involved in pain perception. Coping strategies and cognitive appraisal of a situation also play a role and are believed to cause self-induced release of the pain-attenuating endorphins. Pain comes in many guises. For example, anxiety, feelings of inadequacy, or hostile and aggressive drives can fuel "psychological pain." Often individuals find "relief" from such "pain" with morphine—they fall into the "arms of Morpheus," god of dreams, and son of Hypnos, the god of sleep; hence the term *morphine* to describe the drug's sedative and sleep-promoting effects.

At small to moderate doses, of about five to ten milligrams, morphine can produce the most consummate sense of euphoria with loss of all anxiety. Muscle relaxation occurs, pain is eliminated, and respiration becomes slow. Its ability to reduce sensitivity to both external and internal stimuli leads to loss of concentration and a dreamlike state, which culminates eventually in a calm sleep. Morphine is believed to mediate these effects though its actions in the emotional centers of the brain, such as the amygdala. At slightly higher doses an abnormal state of euphoria occurs, which is quite different from that experienced with lower doses. Injecting heroin, or morphine, into a vein produces a "whole body orgasm," or "rush." At present there is no scientific explanation for this, and in some individuals the opposite effect, *dysphoria*, may occur, which manifests itself as restlessness and anxiety.

With higher doses of morphine, sedation can descend into unconsciousness. The breathing rate becomes depressed, owing to morphine's inhibitory action on the brain centers that trigger respiration. This can lead to death, but the quantities required greatly exceed the average dose used by morphine addicts. Death by "overdose" most often arises from a lack of self-esteem, which drives individuals to the abuse of many drugs mixed with all sorts of adulterants. The rock star Janis Joplin was renowned for her powerful and frenzied performances, but offstage she required heroin and Southern Comfort to alleviate her fears of being unable to sing. On October 4, 1970, she died of an "overdose."

These extraordinary effects of morphine lead inexorably to a compulsive habit. When morphine or heroin is used frequently, the euphoric effects diminish, a tolerance develops, and increasing amounts are required to achieve an effect similar to the initial experience. In time a regular opiate user begins to require doses that would be lethal to a normal individual. More surprising, this chronic opiate use does not cause any appreciable damage to the body. Any damage that arises is caused mainly by the lifestyle of the user that features malnutrition, infection, and neglect for fear that medical examination may reveal their addiction. A higher metabolic rate and more effective elimination can explain tolerance to many drugs, but with opiates it appears that the nerve cells become adapted to its continuing presence. In other words, in the absence of the drug, the cells can no longer function normally.

The opiate withdrawal, or abstinence, syndrome manifests itself as a collection of intense, physical symptoms, which some addicts refer to as "dying sick." The symptoms are the opposite of those experienced on first exposure to morphine. After about two days, the individual cannot sleep and becomes restless and anxious. There is increased sensitivity to pain, and diarrhea accompanied by abdominal cramps occurs—in the past morphine was a life-saving drug in cases of dysentery and diarrhea because its action on the intestine increases water reabsorption and slows digestion. The withdrawal effects are not life-threatening—they are often like a bad dose of flu—and disappear within a few days. The vigor and duration of the withdrawal syndrome relates directly to the duration of previous drug use and the intensity of its effects. For example, withdrawal from heroin results in severe but short-lived effects, whereas with methadone, which is less potent, they are prolonged but not so harsh.

The neurochemical basis for the withdrawal syndrome was not discovered until 1975, when Marshall Nirenberg and colleagues at the National Institutes of Health, in Bethesda, Maryland, showed a relationship between tolerance and dependence using cultured nerve cells. All three types of opiate receptors mediate slow modulatory neurotransmission. This, you may recall, involves the activation or inhibition of a receptor-linked enzyme on the inner face of the nerve cell membrane, which regulates the opening or closing of ion channels from the inside of the cell. Opiates, which are agonists, activate their receptor, resulting in reduced enzyme activity and inhibition of nerve cell firing.

With continued exposure to the opiate, however, the nerve cell compensates by manufacturing increased amounts of the enzyme. In other words, the cell "learns" to operate in the continued presence of the drug—it becomes physically dependent on it. Therefore, when the drug is withdrawn, the activity of the enzyme remains excessively high until the amount of enzyme present returns to the normal level. In the brain this has direct consequences for other neurons, such as those in the locus coeruleus, the rate of firing of which is inhibited by the opioid-containing neurons. The rate of firing in the cells of the locus coeruleus adapts to the continued presence of opiates but becomes significantly reduced in the period immediately following drug withdrawal. This in turn results in loss of inhibitory control of cortical cell firing. The resulting excessive excitation in the cortex may contribute to features of the abstinence syndrome, but precisely how this happens is still unclear.

Too often, however, the world's media would have us believe that we are spiraling rapidly into an opiate epidemic. In reality, much of this is a farrago of myth and anecdotal evidence. We really do not know the size of the problem, because the trade is clandestine, and we can rely only on indirect indicators such as drug seizures, detection of underground laboratories, arrest of drug abusers, and emergency room visits. Still, regular users worldwide are relatively uncommon, at an estimated eight million people or 0.14 percent of the global population. If we lump together all forms of unlawful drugs, the number of users rise to 10 percent of the global population. Yet society continues to reserve a curious form of pharmacological Calvinism for such "illegal" substances while maintaining an ambivalence toward other "legal" forms. Alcohol is consumed by at least half of the global population, and nicotine is used by probably 30 percent, although this latter number is dramatically decreasing.

Eau de Vie—Joie de Vivre

With its beginnings in prehistory, alcohol use most probably arose because ingestion of partially fermented, sugar-rich fruits or grains found favor in many human societies. It is hard to believe that the technological innovations that evolved to improve and increase the production of alcohol were undertaken for the relief of thirst or for its nutritional value. Alcohol is pleasurable; its soporific effects allow us to escape, forget, and explore. The rapid passage of this beguilingly simple, uncharged molecule into the brain brings a unique sense of physical enjoyment. It produces a warm flush to the skin by dilating the blood vessels, enhances social interactions by increasing assertiveness, and relieves the anxieties that generate interpersonal tensions. Should a similar chemical be discovered tomorrow, it would be hailed as a wonder drug.

But alcohol is far from being a stimulant. As the dose increases from one to four milligrams of alcohol to every milliliter of blood, one steadily progresses from being dizzy and delightful to drunk and disorderly to "dead drunk" and in danger of death. The enhanced social interactions initially experienced turn into excessive excitement and even aggression. Self-restraint is lost and coordination of speech and physical movement vanishes. This arises from the sedative effects of alcohol on delicately controlled neural activity in the brain stem. Here the extremely active circuits of the locus coeruleus and raphe nuclei are first affected, and this results in the loss of control in the many regions of the brain to which they send their vine-like axons. This in turn leads to the uncontrolled responses and memory loss that accompanies excessive alcohol use. Indeed, very high concentrations of alcohol can induce a comatose state. The respiratory center in the mid-brain can become paralyzed, and death may ensue.

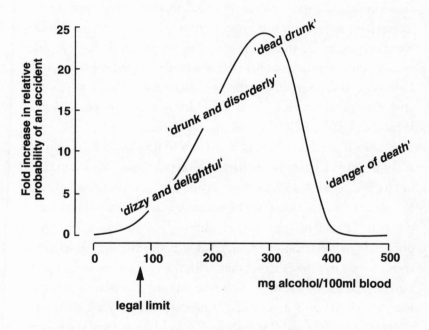

FIGURE 6.2. The dose-response effects of alcohol are illustrated by comparing the frequency of accidents with increasing blood alcohol levels. The legal limit indicates the amount of blood alcohol permitted when driving a vehicle.

However, as with morphine, death by alcohol "overdose" more often than not involves a fatal accident caused by the loss of physical coordination. Less commonly, it can be due to the additional use of sedatives, such as diazepam (Valium), or heroin. Laudanum, for example, was a mix of opium and alcohol; such preparations are often euphemistically termed a *tincture*. Laudanum was the prized drink of the English poet Samuel Taylor Coleridge, who used about four pints a week while writing his rather strange *Rime of the Ancient Mariner*. Some preparations of alcohol may contain a stimulant—absinthe is an example. This pale-green liqueur is made by distilling alcohol in which a variety of herbs have been steeped. Wormwood (*Artemesia absinthium*) is the most important ingredient, because it contains a stimulant called *thujone*. In small amounts absinthe was said to stimulate the mind and the sexual appetite, but in excessive amounts it produced terrifying hallucinations. While it was declared to be the drink of the avant-garde, including nineteenth-century French bohemian artists, de Maupassant, Toulouse Lautrec, and van Gogh, the effects claimed for absinthe were probably due to alcoholism. The legal drink that survives today as Pernod or Ricard lacks the wormwood thujone.

Unlike morphine, there is no known brain receptor for alcohol. Alcohol is an electrically uncharged molecule, and it seeks similarly uncharged regions, such as those inside the membranes of all cells. Cell membranes are made up of molecules, called *phospholipids*, and proteins. The cell membrane is a highly ordered structure. The phospholipids are electrically uncharged at one end, and these uncharged regions tend to associate together, with the charged ends facing the outside and the inside of the cell where molecules bearing complementary electrical charges exist. When viewed with a high-resolution microscope, the cell membrane looks like a railway track—the rails representing the charged parts of the phospholipids, and the ties the uncharged parts. These phospholipids provide a fluid environment; some membranes have the consistency of olive oil. The fluid nature of membranes is essential to the proper functioning of the membrane proteins. The ion channels of brain cell membranes, for example, require a flexible environment to allow them to open and close in response to voltage change or the binding of a neurotransmitter. The electrically uncharged nature of alcohol, therefore, which has a natural affinity for the electrically inert core of the membrane, can disrupt membrane organization and indirectly influence the functioning of the associated ion channels.

In this way, alcohol can alter practically every aspect of nerve cell conduction and neurotransmission. It will slow the shuttling of sodium and potassium ions through their membrane ion channels and reduce nerve cell firing, especially in very active groups of neurons, such as those located in the brain stem. GABA-mediated inhibitory neurotransmission is particularly sensitive to the action of alcohol. There seems to be a site, or "pocket," at which alcohol can influence the action of GABA on its receptor. Like the benzodiazepines, it seems to cause some sort of shape change at the GABA binding site, which results in enhanced conduction of chloride ions into the cell and inhibition of nerve cell firing. This probably explains why the antianxiety and sedative actions of alcohol are not unlike those of the benzodiazepines. By contrast, the memory-impairing actions of alcohol and blockade of LTP arise from its ability to dampen the excitatory effects of glutamate on nerve cell firing. This action of alcohol seems to result mainly from its slowing of the gating of sodium and calcium ions in response to the action of glutamate at its NMDA receptor.

John Barleycorn

Alcohol is not a very potent drug; about a half a milligram in every milliliter of blood is required to experience its euphoric effects. But tolerance develops rapidly, and increasing amounts of alcohol become necessary if its effects are to be maintained. This leads to physical dependence, as the metabolizing enzymes in the liver grow increasingly more effective in their ability to eliminate alcohol. In stark contrast to morphine, the tolerance and physical dependence induced by alcohol can take months or years to develop. Individuals who are physically dependent on alcohol need to consume about 250–300 grams of alcohol per day—at least a bottle of whisky. This leads to physical changes in the brain. The ability of alcohol to enhance neurotransmission at the GABA receptor is lost, because the structure of the receptor becomes changed due to selective suppression of the synthesis of certain parts of the receptor ion channel complex. Conversely, the inhibitory effect of alcohol at the glutamate NMDA receptor results in the increased production of receptors, as the brain struggles to overcome the continued presence of the drug. These changes have considerable consequences for alcohol abstinence syndrome.

A lot of alcohol must be consumed regularly to achieve a state of dependence; nevertheless, many researchers believe that the hangover that follows a night's drinking constitutes an abstinence syndrome. This assumption is based mainly on the relief provided by another drink—the so-called hair-of-the-dog. This view represents only a virtuous principle—it is a reprimand in perfect accord with a chemical crime. However, following withdrawal from significant alcohol abuse—at least a bottle of whisky a day for a period of several weeks—profuse sweating, anxiety, nausea, and vomiting occur within hours. These symptoms are not unlike those that accompany opiate abstinence syndrome because they also arise from excessive firing of nerve cells following their sudden release from the constraining effects of alcohol. The generalized excitability arises from increased glutamate function; the anxiety, sleeplessness, poor mood, and mental discomfort are due to the loss of GABA-mediated inhibition. During the following day or two, these symptoms get worse and can often develop into life-threatening seizures if not treated. Increasing agitation, confusion, and hallucinations, generally referred to as *delirium tremens*, or the "DTs," continue over the next two to four days. The occurrence of hallucinations probably relates to altered nerve cell activity in the raphe nucleus, as the hallucinations produced by LSD arise from its effects in this region of the brain. The magnitude of alcohol abstinence syndrome can best be understood by reading Jack London's autobiographical novel *John Barleycorn*.

Alcohol's lack of potency has another cost: the need to employ large quantities of the drug places a heavy burden on the body. The liver, which metabolizes and eliminates the alcohol from the body, is particularly sensitive. Here an enzyme (alcohol dehydrogenase) transforms the alcohol into acetaldehyde. Since this is quite toxic, another enzyme (aldehyde dehydrogenase) quickly converts it to acetate, which is a rich and ready source of calories, about 100 calories per drink. The effects of continued alcohol metabolism on the liver are twofold. First, it stimulates the synthesis of fatty acids, which leads to what is termed a "fatty liver." This condition is benign, but, after years of alcohol abuse, it can develop into a lethal condition called alcoholic hepatitis. This is characterized by the cell death and organ inflammation that precede liver cirrhosis. Second, the toxicity of the acetaldehyde that is generated during alcohol metabolism further contributes to liver cell death.

The harmful effects of alcohol on the brain are more difficult to evaluate. The cognitive deficits associated with excessive alcohol use are small and inconsistent, and the brain shrinkage observed in some alcoholics does not seem to be due to brain cell loss. The problem here is that many of these studies are retrospective, and, as a result, it is almost impossible to separate the direct and indirect effects of alcohol. The direct effects of alcohol may relate to altered protein synthesis, since this would impair the general maintenance of nerve cells involved in cognitive processes. This would explain why the reported physical changes reverse upon abstinence from alcohol, the exception being the memory capacity that is reliant on the hippocampus, arguably the most dynamic region required for learning. The indirect effects of alcohol abuse arise from falls, fights, and car accidents. The cumulative effects of malnutrition, vitamin loss, and general incapacitation of the liver render the heavy drinker vulnerable to serious brain damage. A condition called Wernicke's syndrome is due to thiamine deficiency and, unless treated with vitamin replacement therapy, it can develop into Korsakoff's syndrome, in which the damage to the brain becomes irreversible. With Korsakoff's syndrome the individual is completely disorientated and tends to fabricate imaginary experiences in compensation for the loss of memory.

Chemical Cures for Angst

Despite its risky side effects, humans have always considered alcohol to be a wonder drug, the "water of life"—*eau de vie* in French, or *uisce beatha* in Gaelic. For centuries the euphoric qualities of this anodyne have served as a relief for anxiety, that unsettling apprehension and uncertainty that all of us feel to some degree. But in moderation, anxiety is actually a very good thing. The Manhattan angst of Woody Allen was the creative fulcrum for his entire movie *oeuvre*. It is an important force in human affairs. In my view, people who are perfectly tranquil and unruffled are not likely to be interesting, motivated, or creative, which are key elements in successfully attaining our goals and desires.

Like pain, anxiety has great survival value—it triggers the "fight or flight" response. For some people, however, anxiety is a crippling obstacle that prevents them from achieving their goals. Depending on how it is defined, severe anxiety is remarkably common, affecting between 5 and 10 percent of the world's population. Phobias, for example, can range from a simple fear of snakes and spiders to fear of scrutiny by one's peers to a feeling of being unable to escape from a seemingly innocuous situation. Phobias can manifest as continuing and excessive worry, or obsessive and compulsive habits that are believed to allay the underlying anxiety. In its most severe form, however, anxiety can lead to absolute terror and panic accompanied by trembling, heart palpitations, and feelings of being smothered. It is not surprising that many of these individuals also suffer from alcoholism. Psychotherapy is the preferred means of treating anxiety, but, more often than not, antianxiety drugs, which give fast and effective relief without eliminating the underlying cause, are used to treat it.

In the mid-nineteenth century the German chemist Adolph von Baeyer synthesised barbituric acid. Although inactive, it provided the chemical skeleton that Fischer and von Mehring used to produce the first sedatives—barbitone, in 1903, and phenobarbitone, in 1912. These became instantly popular as drugs that facilitated sleep and produced antianxiety effects when taken during the daytime. They also proved to be effective agents in the treatment of epilepsy. Like all agents that allay anxiety, the demand for these agents was extraordinary. In the mid-1930s whole arrays of new barbiturates were developed—long-acting forms, short-acting forms, and forms that could be used for intravenous anaesthesia. Over 2,500 different barbiturates were synthesized, and fifty reached the market. By the mid-1960s, 500 tons of barbiturates were being synthesized annually, enough for forty to fifty doses for every man, woman, and child in the United States alone. Unfortunately, like alcohol, they produced tolerance and a physical dependence, which was due largely to their ability to activate the liver enzymes involved in their degradation. The potent sedative action of barbiturates gave them the unenviable reputation of being the drugs most frequently used for suicide. It was acute barbiturate intoxication that caused the untimely demise of Marilyn Monroe.

Clearly, something other than a "sleeping pill" was required for the treatment of anxiety. The first move in this direction was serendipitous. In the mid-1940s Frank Berger, a Czechoslovakian chemist then working in London on a series of antibacterial agents, noted a compound with remarkable muscle-relaxing properties. This observation led to the development of mephenesin for the treatment of painful muscle contractions, such as those arising from the displacement of a disc in the vertebral column. But mephenesin had another effect in these patients—it seemed to ease their anxiety without making them drowsy.

This was an important observation because it heralded the idea that a drug could have selective effects on anxiety. This led to the development of a related compound, meprobamate, which was promoted as a more selective antianxiety drug than barbiturates. The challenge to enter this lucrative market with an even more selective antianxiety agent was taken up by the Roche drug company. Since nobody really knew how mephenesin produced its effects, they screened drugs at random, searching for antianxiety action in mice and rats. One of the Roche researchers, Leo Sternbach, had a particular interest in a group of chemical compounds that were unrelated to any known sedative. Not surprising, they had no antianxiety effects, and they were about to be set aside when a final compound was sent for testing. It proved to be a most effective antianxiety agent. Its structure had been wrongly identified—it was benzodiazepine chlordiazepoxide.

By 1960 chlordiazepoxide (Librium) was on the market and competing with meprobamate (Miltown). Diazepam (Valium) followed in 1963. The era of Librium and Valium was born. Sales rose rapidly, and by the mid-1970s benzodiazepines were the most commonly prescribed drugs. Benzodiazepines came to be regarded as panaceas, too often employed in the absence of genuine anxiety. They were used simply to help in coping with everyday life. Their indiscriminate use is now curtailed, but benzodiazepines still remain among the most frequently prescribed drugs.

Benzodiazepines have a specific action in the brain. They bind to

TABLE 6.1 Drugs Used to Treat Anxiety

Agent	Transmitter affected
Barbiturates	
Pentobarbitone Phenobarbitone } Thiopentone	Enhance the action of GABA
Benzodiazepines	
Chlordiazepoxide Diazepam Clonazepam } Flunitrazepam Temazepam	Enhance the action of GABA

Although the benzodiazepines are the drugs of choice for the treatment of anxiety, the barbiturates may still be used in the treatment of epilepsy (phenobarbitone) and as intravenous anaesthetics (thiopentone). It should also be noted that the benzodiazepines and barbiturates act at different sites on the GABA recptor.

a site on the GABA receptor complex. When benzodiazepine is present, the GABA transmitter can bind more effectively to its receptor, and the net result is increased gating of chloride ions into the cell, hyperpolarization, and a decreased firing rate. In other words, they indirectly have the effects of drugs that are agonists at the GABA receptor. The action of the benzodiazepines proved to be much more specific than that of the barbiturates. Their influence is directed more toward brain areas involved in the modulation of emotion, fear, and aggression, especially the amygdala. Thus, unlike the generalized action of barbiturates, which affects areas of the brain stem that regulate awareness and wakefulness, benzodiazepines are specific and truly effective antianxiety agents.

However, the rather specific action of benzodiazepines in the amygdala and hippocampus has a drawback. Owing to the complex roles of these brain regions in processing information for long-term memory, it is not surprising to find that benzodiazepines can cause amnesia. The impairment depends on the dose and applies only to the recall of events that occur while the drug is present. This is one of the reasons for their use in minor surgical procedures. But the most remarkable feature of benzodiazepines is that they are safer than barbiturates. Overdoses of more than a hundred pills have been reported to have effects no worse than three days' continuous sleep. Why benzodiazepine receptors exist in the brain still remains a mystery. It is possible that a chemical system with effects analogous to those of benzodiazepines exists in the brain to control our states of anxiety, and a group of possible transmitters, known as the *beta-carbolines*, has been suggested to play such a role. However, their biochemical pathways and physiological functions are still unclear.

Dopamine Dollars

The perspective on drug action outlined above is overly simplistic because it fails to explain the elusive condition constantly referred to as a "sense of euphoria." Why does the brain "value" the actions of drugs such as heroin, alcohol, or barbiturates yet place such little worth on benzodiazepines? Is it possible to describe the chemical currency of pleasure? Some scientists believe we can. Their arguments are based on the belief that these drugs act on a neural pathway that provides us with a sensation of pleasure, an evolutionarily conserved system that drives all organisms toward inwardly rewarding stimuli, such as food and sex.

Research in the mid-1950s demonstrated the existence of a reward center in the brain. This region is known as the *nucleus accumbens*. Located deep in the forebrain, it is connected to the nearby amygdala and hippocampus, which lie against the overlying *temporal cortex*. Importantly, the nucleus accumbens receives axons from nerve cells in the brain stem, the ventral tegmental area, that use dopamine as a neurotransmitter. If an animal is allowed to press a lever that results in the electrical stimulation of this brain circuit, it quickly learns to repeat this task with increasing frequency. In other words, the surge of dopamine released by stimulation provides a reward that positively reinforces the learning of the task.

Direct pharmacological evidence for the role of dopamine in the sensation of pleasure is provided by a self-administration procedure that allows the injection of drugs into the bloodstream, or directly into the brain circuit, through a permanent catheter, or tube. In this case, pressing a lever causes a pump to deliver controlled amounts of a drug. Drugs that are dopamine agonists positively reinforce lever-pressing, whereas dopamine antagonists do not. These observations suggest that the nerve cell pathway from the ventral tegmental area to the nucleus accumbens forms the "pleasure center," and dopamine is the "pleasure currency" of the brain.

All abuse-prone drugs exert some effect in this reward circuit of the brain. Animals learn quickly to self-administer such drugs with increasing frequency. The list is comprehensive, for it includes virtually every drug used for its pleasurable effects. Morphine, alcohol, barbiturates, amphetamines, nicotine, and caffeine all positively reinforce the task of lever pressing; that is, the animal will continuously press a lever in order to receive the drug. Not all of these drugs reinforce the behavior, nor is the pattern of self-administration always the same, but they are all drugs that are self-administered by humans. The ability of these agents to release dopamine in the reward circuit may seem surprising given that they all have very different modes of action. The effect is obvious for substances such as amphetamine or cocaine, which enhance dopamine release, but not so apparent for alcohol, which could be expected to decrease dopamine release.

A bigger problem with the idea of dopamine as the "pleasure currency" of the brain is that it leads to the prediction that all drugs capable of elevating this neurotransmitter should be addictive. This, however, is not the case. Deprenyl, which inhibits monoamine oxidase, an enzyme that degrades dopamine, is not addictive and has no reinforcement potential. There must therefore be some other aspect that dictates drug-abuse potential. Environmental factors may play a role. The relative potency of antianxiety drugs could be expected to lead to abuse, yet benzodiazepines have a weak reinforcing potential, and their potent antianxiety effects are not greatly abused. The quest for novelty, such as behaviors associated with thrill seeking or the desire for exploration, may be another factor. Such behaviors have been linked to addiction tendencies in animals, but there is only limited evidence that this link is mediated by dopamine. The idea of drug abuse being related to effects on the brain's reward center is rather clichéd. What really matters is whether a drug causes one compulsively to seek its use. This is often referred to as a *craving*, and it outlives physical dependence by months.

Craving is the kernel of drug addiction. Dramatic physical withdrawal symptoms are not a problem because they are short-lived and easily managed with appropriate medication. Furthermore, the most addictive and dangerous drugs, such as cocaine and methamphetamine, do not produce any notable physical symptoms on withdrawal. While the immediate effects of all addictive drugs may be due to increased dopamine activity in the nucleus accumbens, their prolonged use must result in a persistent change that makes the addicted brain distinctly different from the nonaddicted brain. Indeed, much of the current thinking about dopamine's role in learning and motivation has been influenced by the view that the nucleus accumbens serves as a critical interface between the areas that control emotion and those that control our response to it. It is a system that drives our wants or desires into a behavioral response that becomes stereotyped in our brain and allows us successfully to repeat it in order to satisfy bodily need.

This bodily response becomes part of us; we become psychologically dependent on it. In many ways, our response to an addictive drug can be the same. We develop a strong compulsion or desire to experience the drug's pleasurable effects once more, a psychological dependence that culminates in the habitual use of the drug. The consequence is physical dependence on the drug and a withdrawal syndrome in its absence. Moreover, this physical dependence on the drug leads to another form of psychological dependence. We begin to anticipate the pleasurable consequences of its use and the disadvantages of its absence. These secondary forms of psychological dependence are reinforced by many subtle behavioral stimuli such as the sight or smell of the drug—the open whiskey decanter or the plume of tobacco smoke—and the environmental context of its previously pleasurable effects—even a cup of coffee after a particularly sumptuous meal.

The Blot on the Brain

Some drugs can be so exciting emotionally that they almost leave a scar on the cerebral tissue, an indelible memory that leads one compulsively to seek out that experience again. This must be somehow permanently recorded in the brain. Genetic influences are believed to be important in determining our sensitivity to drugs. The finding of a strong association between a gene that encodes a particular form of the dopamine receptor and alcoholism has received much attention, given the importance of dopamine in the rewarding effects of alcohol. But this association does not appear to be specific to alcoholism, since the same gene has been found in conditions such as attention deficit hyperactivity disorder, posttraumatic stress disorder, and autism, all conditions that are not necessarily associated with substance abuse. Genes do not determine anything; they may indicate a predisposition to substance abuse, but most drug users do not become drug abusers, or even drug dependent.

As described above, continuing exposure to morphine or alcohol results in gradual adaptations of the brain through altered gene expression and signaling between nerve cells. Many of these adaptations can account for the development of tolerance, physical dependence, and a withdrawal syndrome. By contrast, continued exposure to amphetamines, cocaine, or caffeine does not appear to result in significant physical changes in brain structure, a distinction that may ultimately explain why such drugs lack a profound physical withdrawal syndrome. These drugs, however, may activate brain regions other than the reward center and so produce long-lasting drug craving. Whole brain scans of cocaine addicts, for example, show that the amygdala becomes highly excited when the subject is shown a syringe—this has become a secondary reinforcer of pending drug pleasure.

Behavioral changes also occur. Morphine generally impairs the learning and memory processes necessary for the acquisition and retention of some, but not all, associations, and this can greatly affect social behaviour. For example, the ability of morphine to suppress the attention-seeking cries and flailing limb movements of the newborn infant puts at risk the development of early bonding. Equally, driving a car under the influence of alcohol can be erratic at first, but with repeated exposures simple skill adjustments are learned. Such compensation is a form of behavioral tolerance.

Coda

The fact that monkeys readily learn to self-inject addictive drugs, such as morphine, raises another rather interesting issue about the abuse of psychoactive drugs in our society. This observation would seem to imply that drug use is a normal behaviour restrained in humans by social values and customs. It would appear that people who adhere firmly to the ideologies of many religious denominations use less alcohol compared with those whose convictions are not so fervent. Most people consider drug abuse to be an abnormal behavior, and addiction a social problem to be solved by the penal code.

However, this view depends to a large extent on the social context of the drug in question—some societies approve the use of addictive substances such as alcohol, cannabis, and tobacco. Yet the most benevolent view that our own society presently offers is that drug addicts are victims of their social situation—negative family influences, inappropriate peer influence, and temptations to seek sensation or novelty, to name a few. More commonly, drug addicts are considered to be weak and unwholesome individuals incapable of resisting or unwilling to control their own selfish gratification, and even undeserving of treatment. This stigma attached to the addict is far from the truth.

An addicted brain is distinctly different from a nonaddicted brain. Its metabolic activity, receptor sensitivity, and responsiveness to environmental cues are profoundly changed. Is addiction like other chronic relapsing illnesses, such as diabetes or hypertension?

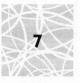

Making Memory

Addiction provides an example of how drugs can alter the basic functioning of the brain. Many of these functional changes appear to be irreversible and have long-lasting consequences for former drug addicts. The amygdala, for example, continues to respond to drug cues, such as the sight of a syringe, long after the addict has overcome the physical effects of drug withdrawal. And we still do not know if drug-induced change in brain function ever returns to the original state. Former alcoholics seem to require the continued reinforcement of abstinence over a lifetime from support groups like Alcoholics Anonymous. This raises the question of how memory is conveyed and sustained. We generally think of memory as an individual faculty. But it is now known that there are multiple memory systems in the brain, each devoted to different memory functions.

The Sketchpad of the Mind

We are built to process stimuli, to seek out and analyze those that are important to us, to produce new perceptions, and, ultimately, to alter our ways of looking at the world. To do this we must keep in "mind" concepts, ideas, or schemes and compare them with what we "know" of our previous experiences and memories. This is known as *working memory*. Alan Baddeley, an English psychologist at the University of Cambridge, who introduced the concept in the mid-1970s, termed working memory our "executive function." Many refer to working memory as short-term memory, but it is much more than that: it is an active processing system, a mechanism we use in our thinking and reasoning. It is our awareness. Baddeley used a lovely metaphor for working memory: he described it as our mental "sketchpad," implying that it had both limited capacity and erasibility.

Working memory is what we think about or pay attention to. For example, the sensory systems of our brain, such as those associated with hearing or seeing, constantly receive information—a sort of immediate memory that can fade away in milliseconds. The capacity of our immediate memory is small, allowing us to store around seven items, such as numbers, at any given time. We make a telephone call by holding "in mind" the number before dialing it. But immediate memory can be prolonged when it becomes matched with information stored as long-term memory. This is where working memory comes into play: it serves to hold recent information "online," while it is compared with and referenced to information already stored. In this manner working memory can extend the lifetime of immediate memory into minutes, or even longer should we wish to commit the information to long-term memory.

Working memory is the brain's "knowing" system. It allows our internal representations of the world, encoded in our nerve cells, to interact with the external signals that guide our behavior. These provide us with the experiences we use to modify our internal representations. Working memory is highly developed in humans, who are unique in their use of structured language. When we converse with someone, our working memory holds segments of the other person's speech for several seconds, while continuing to receive the next segment of words for subsequent scanning. This aspect of working memory may have been a critical factor in the evolution and definition of human intelligence.

Where and how does the brain evaluate temporary information? In the late 1930s it was observed that damage to frontal lobes of the brain, especially in a region called the *prefrontal cortex*, prevented monkeys from retaining temporary information necessary to carry out a particular task. The experimental task employed then is now referred to as the *delayed-response test*. In this task the monkey watches an experimenter place a food reward into one of two wells, which are then covered with different objects, such as a colored cube or cylinder. There is then a delay period, during which a screen is lowered to block the view, before the monkey's accuracy in retrieving the reward is determined. The monkey has to remember that the reward is under a specific object, not simply any object. When the prefrontal cortex is damaged, the monkey persistently fails to make the correct selection despite remaining perfectly capable of carrying out other complex tasks.

It seems that the prefrontal cortex has the capacity to "know" that an object exists in time and space, even when it is not in view. Using tasks similar to the delayed-response test, Patricia Goldman-Rakic, an American neurobiologist at Yale University, has now identified a specific group of nerve cells in the prefrontal cortex that activate only during the delay period and at no other time during the task. Although this does not explain the mechanism of working memory, it identifies at least one possible site for working memory—a place where we keep information "in mind" for immediate use.

Not only are the prefrontal lobes important in relating our internal and external environments, they may also play a bigger role in forming our personality. Take, for example, the unfortunate case of Phineas Gage. In the mid-1800s Gage was a foreman overseeing blasting work at a railway construction site in Vermont. While packing explosive into a borehole, his attention was diverted, and the tamping iron hit the rock and sparked the dynamite, which blasted the huge spear of the tamping iron straight through his head. It entered just below his left eyesocket, passed through the prefrontal lobe, and exited at the top of his cranium. Despite the considerable infection that followed, he recovered. His personality, however, had irrevocably changed. He was no longer the reliable foreman of the past; he had become erratic and undependable, impatient and without restraint. In the view of his colleagues, Gage simply was "no longer Gage."

The Vaults of the Brain

We now know much more about how short-term, or working memory, is converted into long-term memory. It was the Canadian psychologist Donald Hebb, in the late 1940s, who postulated that long-term memory was retained in specific brain areas by an increased excitability that led to the strengthening of synaptic connections between the component nerve cells. In the mid-1970s Tim Bliss and Terje Lømo, then working at the University of Oslo in Norway, provided the evidence. After driving an electrical current into one group of nerve cells, they found that the group they influenced increased in excitability. Only the stimulated nerve cell responded, and the increased excitability did not spread in an arbitrary fashion. More important, the synaptic response outlived the initial stimulus by hours, days, and even weeks. As described in chapter 4, this phenomenon is now known as LTP, and its enduring, rather than fleeting, nature has all the characteristics that are necessary for the construction of memories. But if our memories are to remain, then some physical change must occur—memory cannot be imprinted on molecules since molecules are constantly rejuvenated by the body at different rates.

The study of behavior in sea slugs (*Aplysia californica*) has provided us with important insights into how experience can modify neural pathways. Because the nervous system of the sea slug contains only a few dozen neurons, learning-induced change, such as the persistent withdrawal of the gill in response to an irritating stimulus, can be studied in individual nerve cells. This response requires the formation of many new synaptic contacts in the brain pathways that control gill withdrawal. More important, this research has demonstrated gene activation to be the fundamental prerequisite for translating enduring neural activity into physical change in the nervous system. Gene activation leads to the synthesis of proteins necessary for the structural change that is initiated by dendritic growth and culminates in new synapse formation.

When a drug that activates the glutamate receptor is added to cultured nerve cells in the laboratory, a remarkable response occurs within one to two minutes. From the surface of the nerve cells, myriad finger-like extensions miraculously appear, constantly changing their shape and position like tiny wriggling sacks—a muddling mass of dendrites bobbing all over the place. While they are elegant and fascinating to watch, it is hard to believe that this happens in our brain every time we need to store memory. In the brain neurons are tightly packed together with glia filling every space and closely surrounding every synapse. Yet, despite this complexity, the most consistently reported consequence of learning is change in synapse number. This has been observed in all species and with all models of memory, including LTP. Moreover, learning-induced change in synapse number is a special characteristic of the hippocampus, a brain region intimately involved in processing information for long-term memory.

So how do new dendrites redefine the order, or connectivity pattern, of the existing synapses? A possible answer to this question concerns a group of proteins called *cell adhesion molecules*. These proteins are found on the surface of every cell in the body, and, as their name implies, they seem to dictate how cells behave with one another. These cell adhesion molecules act as social organizers; they determine which cells will group together, and one of their functions in the brain is to maintain contact at synapses. During the period of increased neural activity that immediately follows learning, or LTP, these cell adhesion molecules are stripped from the nerve cell surface, and, as a consequence, the contacts made by the existing synapses are weakened. The weakened synapses provide an opportunity for the new dendrites to eliminate the older synapses and build a new pattern of connectivity. The new dendrites are produced many hours later, and newly synthesized cell adhesion molecules grow, dotting the perimeter of the new synapses, and serve to "glue" them into place. But not all of these new synapses are retained—the brain does not have the capacity for unlimited growth. Useless synapses become lost over time, and only those necessary for memory are retained.

The construction of neural circuits in response to experience takes time. An animal trained to perform a task just before surgical removal of its hippocampus will have no recall of that task at any time following surgery. However, if a critical period of time is allowed to elapse between training and surgery, then perfect recall is retained. This critical period is about four days in the rat, four weeks in the primate, and up to one or two decades in humans. So where does the information relocate? The cortex is believed to be the final repository for the long-term storage of our memories. Nerve cell pathways connect the cortex to the hippocampus. These pathways are bidirectional and allow the reciprocal exchange of information. Learning in the hippocampus is fast and fleeting; it constantly instructs the cortex, the education of which is slow but enduring. The placement of memory is a rather circumspect process. Synapse number change in the hippocampus is large but transient; that in the cortex is small but long-lasting.

A Blueprint for the Brain

The relative size of brain-to-body weight is surprisingly constant among mammals; the ratio is precisely the same for both the elephant and the shrew. The size of the cortex, or those regions that control movement, is also constant when compared to the size of the whole brain. It would seem that genetic instructions for the blueprint of the brain have been conserved during mammalian evolution. This makes good sense. If one part of the brain enlarges, then the size of those parts that work with it may be expected to show a corresponding change in size. But this does not mean that brains are alike in every way. Uniformity allows one to view general features of brain organization, but when examined more closely, an impressive array of specialization exists between species.

Major regions of the mammalian brain are organized for receiving and analyzing information. There are at least a dozen areas in the visual cortex of the brain that respond differently to the attributes of an object, such as its color, size, or movement. The unique use of language by humans is reflected in the development of specific brain regions. Learning a foreign language in adulthood employs a brain area that is distinct from that used in establishing one's first language. Communication by speech is particularly dependent on working memory, for which the prefrontal lobe has been significantly enlarged. Environmental instructions, however, determine how the nerve cell pathways of these regions will be formed, the nature and use of their synaptic connections, and the extent to which they are stimulated by surrounding circumstances. Unstimulated nerve cells simply die, while unused synapses disappear. Cell death is an important phenomenon in the construction of the mature nervous system, a kind of editing of unnecessary connections.

But experience continues to tune this rough-and-ready apparatus for its precise job. The cortical regions that receive and process information are not static—they can change. Learning can lead to structural alterations in the brain. There appears to be use-dependent competition for cortical territory. The cortical areas that control our movements change as we acquire new skills; they modify their circuits, and, should the skill require new circuits, they encroach on adjacent cortical areas. The architecture of every brain is individually modified because we exercise our skills in different ways. This is the biological basis for experience: it is related to our capacity to know the external world, and it is the biology of human intelligence.

8

The Lost Truth and Its Restitution

The Illusory Milieu

The translation of experiences into memories seems to occur through a series of events in which enduring neural activity, driven by a bath of ever-changing chemicals, causes the physical alteration of brain structure. Drugs may interact with this bath of chemicals to alter how we process information (recall that caffeine enhances LTP) and have a significant influence on the nature of the memory that is stored. This raises an interesting issue when we consider the drugs used to treat depression and schizophrenia. These are debilitating conditions in which thought and emotion are severely disturbed; they are frightening, not only for the sufferer but also the caregiver, who often cannot accept the bizarre behavior of a loved one. Is there some brain region in which a physiological and functional basis for this vulnerability might be found? Temporal lobe epilepsy is a condition in which brain seizures occur in the temporal lobe, the part of the cortex that contains the hippocampus and amygdala. Individuals who suffer such seizures frequently report intense emotion and paranoia. They fear being in a strange or unreal state. They may even experience "revelations of truth." The temporal lobe, that great modulator of human behavior, may be the place where the unconscious resurges into the conscious. Is it then possible that drugs can also alter the altered mind?

Classifying the symptoms of depression or schizophrenia is no easy matter. Consider the history of the *Diagnostic and Statistical Manual of Mental Disorders* (*DSM*), the reference manual that resides on the shelf of every practicing psychiatrist. This is the American Psychiatric Association's 900-page guide for the description and classification of mental disorders, including depression and schizophrenia. The forerunner of this manual, published in 1918, went through ten editions before *DSM-I* was published in 1952. *DSM-II* followed in 1968, a small spiral-bound notebook of less than 150 pages. The reasons for revising *DSM-II* were manifold, not least because it included homosexuality as a mental disorder. *DSM-III* appeared in 1980, and a revised version in 1983 (*DSM-III-R*). Over half the diagnostic categories were changed, and thirty new diagnostic categories were added. Some so-called disorders, such as premenstrual dysphoric disorder, were excluded because they were regarded as having negative implications for women. Eventually, in 1994, *DSM-IV* was published, the work of 1,000 acknowledged consultants.

Over this short space of time the number of categories of mental illness steadily increased: *DSM-II* described some 180 disorders; this number increased to 292 in *DSM-III-R*, and *DSM-IV* has over 350 categories. This blossoming of categories serves to demonstrate that our basic understanding of mental illness is poor, or even misguided. Some investigators, such as the American psychiatrists Nancy Andreasen, at the University of Iowa, and Kay Jamison, at Johns Hopkins University, have studied the basis of creativity in the hope that an understanding of this unique thought process may provide insight into the prevalence of mood disorders in artists.

It is worthwhile to consider at the outset these words in honor of the American poet Robert Lowell, written by Irish poet and winner of the Nobel Prize in literature Seamus Heaney. In this passage

Heaney describes the nature of Lowell's extraordinary creative ability. This description is relevant to the subject at hand because Lowell suffered from manic depression.

> [He] had in awesome abundance the poet's first gift for surrender to those energies of language that heave to the fore matter that will not be otherwise summoned, or that might be otherwise suppressed. Under the ray of his concentration, the molten stuff of the psyche ran hot and unstaunched. But its final form was as much beaten as poured, the cooling ingot was assiduously hammered. A fully human and relentless intelligence was at work upon the pleasuring quick of the creative act. He was and will remain a pattern for poets in his amphibiousness, this ability to plunge into the downward reptilian welter of the individual self and yet raise himself with whatever knowledge he gained there out on the hard ledges of the historical present.*

From this passage it would seem that creative people seek to isolate themselves in a manner allowing for the expression of unconscious thoughts and processes that would otherwise be censored by the reality of their surroundings—the psychiatrist would call this a "state of dissociation." They seem to slip into other states of consciousness, where they may remain for hours, sorting through disparate concepts or forms that are initially abstract, but which gradually generate the cohesive concept that finally emerges. Creativity, therefore, does not appear to be logical or rational; it cannot be consciously planned or willed into existence. Rather it is mystical and almost transcendental in nature.

Outwardly, creative people are also different from a behavioral

---

* Heaney, S., "Robert Lowell: A Memorial Address," *Agenda* (Robert Lowell special issue) 18 (1980): 26.

point of view. They are rebellious but retain sensitivity, exploratory in a way that pushes at the limits of social norms, curious to move into the domains of the mind that conventional society perceives as hidden or forbidden. They approach the world without preconceptions, and they pursue their ideas with an obstinate perseverance until they are perfected. These characteristics tend to isolate them from society and can lead to feelings of alienation or loneliness. These personality traits may explain vulnerability to fluctuations in mood. Creative individuals, such as musicians, poets and novelists, or visual artists, are eighteen times more likely to commit suicide and ten times more likely to suffer from depression. This connection needs to be tested more rigorously. Nevertheless, creativity is not incompatible with occasional bouts of "madness," while, at the same time, artistic works can be perfectly lucid. After all, sporadic periods of hypertension do not preclude a normal, healthy life.

The Sadness of Fear

All of us are familiar with moods. We can be content, optimistic, or even gregarious; at other times we can be sad, antisocial, or dissatisfied with the world around us. For most individuals these states are usually transient. Mood has an evolutionary value. It structures our personal relationships. We pine in the absence of loved ones, and sometimes we follow impulsive and optimistic leaders. Yet the utility of ordinary sadness and grief is not so obvious, despite their being aroused by the same kinds of losses in almost everyone. Perhaps low mood motivates us to avoid situations that might cause further loss. For example, it could result in altered behavioral strategies, such as submissive behavior following loss of status. Equally, mood can be destructive. Excessive and chronic depression can result in suicide and frenzied mania. Depressed mood often leads to poor judgement in relationships within society, and such conditions are often referred to as "disorders of affect."

Irrespective of any particular culture, 2 to 5 percent of the global population suffer from mood disorders. We really do not have clear definitions for depression, and, in many ways, those that do exist have only a descriptive value. Major depression is probably not a single illness but a group of disorders characterized by an overwhelming sense of sadness, not always with an obvious cause. An inability to concentrate—as if one's thoughts and actions are slowed—insomnia, anorexia, and feelings of hopelessness and guilt often accompany depression. More than sadness, some individuals describe an intense mental "pain," a mood change that robs them of any ability to experience pleasure.

Episodes of major depression recur with intervening periods of normal mood, but, if untreated, these episodes can last for four to twelve months. Mania is the opposite condition. Elation, boundless energy, and optimism are the hallmarks of a manic individual, but, like depression, these symptoms can vary in their intensity. During periods of excessive excitement, manic individuals can become wildly extravagant; they often go on ill-advised spending sprees, become scandalously promiscuous, or have an incessant interest in particular ideas. In this state, which is usually shorter than the periods of depression, they jeopardize their family and work relationships.

If there is one classification of affective disorders that has proved useful, it is the distinction drawn between individuals suffering from depression alone, termed *unipolar depression*, and depression interspersed with periods of mania, termed *bipolar depression*. This distinction comes from studying the incidence of affective disorders in the families of afflicted individuals. For example, Winston Churchill suffered depression, which he referred to as his "black dog," and the recurring incidence of this condition can be traced back in his family at least to the first Duke of Marlborough, who lived in the seventeenth century.

More recent studies indicate that first relatives of individuals who suffer from bipolar depression have a 19 percent risk of suffering from the same condition. For unipolar depression, the risk to first relatives is 10 percent. This genetic predisposition is not absolute, as the probability of identical twins experiencing the same depressive symptoms is only around 50 percent. Since identical twins come from the same fertilized egg and, therefore, have identical genes, we would expect the incidence of the condition to be exactly the same in each twin if depression were dictated by inheritance alone. Such family studies of mania and depression provide the strongest reasons for believing that environmental factors are of great importance. Bipolar individuals, who are usually more disabled and wretched, tend to become ill at an earlier stage than those suffering from unipolar depression. The contributing environmental factors have not yet been pinpointed, but they have been thought to include aspects of childhood, such as the quality of maternal relationships. But these influences may play only a part in shaping our personalities, since they do not seem to predispose people to depression in later life.

Despite these clear distinctions between unipolar and bipolar depression, we still do not understand their biological differences, let alone the brain areas that may be dysfunctional. Basic neuropathological studies on postmortem brain tissue from patients who were depressed are scarce. But the advent of modern brain scanning techniques is beginning to reveal some subtle abnormalities in brain function between patients with these conditions and with nondepressed patients. Cognitive neuroscience is advancing to a stage where it is possible to be quite specific in analyzing neural activity in discrete brain regions. PET (positron emission tomography) scans, a technique that detects region-specific changes in blood flow as a measure of neural activity, have revealed excessive activity in the left amygdala of depressed patients. Also, neural activity in a specific area in the left prefrontal cortex is found to be increased during depression but not in the intervening phase of remission. In bipolar depression a decrease in the neural activity of the left prefrontal lobe is often found. This helps to confirm that unipolar and bipolar depression are separate entities.

These findings point to the hallmark of depression. An overactive amygdala may negatively label the emotional content of experiences and lead to an overwhelming sense of sadness. Alternatively, by attaching no positive label at all, it may result in an inability to sense the pleasurable aspects of experience.

It is likely that the increased activity observed in PET scans of the left prefrontal cortex influences the amygdala because nerve cell pathways are known to interconnect these two brain regions. The potential of the prefrontal cortex to influence the amygdala may give rise to the depressive preoccupations often described by sufferers as intrusive and exceedingly difficult to discontinue. Similar increases in the neural activity of the left prefrontal cortex are seen in individuals asked to ruminate on sad thoughts. Similar approaches have been used to investigate why rates of depression are about twice as high in women as in men. Both sexes show an equal increase in activity in the prefrontal lobe, but the activity in that region of the amygdala is about eight times higher in women. Other environmental factors may be involved, however, with hormonal influence an obvious possibility. Yet, remarkably, there is little information on how environmental factors may alter the progression of mood disorders.

The Fragmented Mind

Originally, the term *schizophrenia* was coined by the Swiss psychiatrist Eugen Bleuler, in the early 1900s, to emphasize that the thoughts and emotions of sufferers had become fragmented, that they were no longer capable of associating their internal representations of the world with reality. This is not a "split personality," a term often used in common parlance to describe schizophrenia. Rather, it is an incapacitating condition of devastating proportions. The symptoms of schizophrenia can be so bizarre that students first coming across the condition are left incredulous. At their first encounter with individuals suffering from schizophrenia, my students often come upon an individual not unlike themselves—for its onset occurs in late adolescence—wearing designer clothes and the latest hairstyle. This individual is willing to engage them in conversation and tell his or her story. But as the tale unfolds, the students invariably begin to consider the story a hoax that the psychiatrist and I have fabricated in collusion with an actor posing as the "patient."

For those suffering from schizophrenia will tell them bizarre yarns: of communing with the divine; of a television presenter who speaks to them directly with veiled threats to their life; of their deformed nose and their wish to remove it; of a voice that directs them to commit murder. All are fictions told with conviction, for they are the "reality" of the individual's life. Yet this is only one form of schizophrenia, often referred to as the *florid state with positive symptoms* (this term has always been a paradox to me). There is another form of schizophrenia, which is characterized by inappropriate emotional responses. Sufferers are often fearful of others, withdrawn, and lack spontaneous speech. They can laugh or cry at the most inappropriate moments or assume, and maintain, the most abnormal postures. Generally speaking, these are features of emotional withdrawal, or "flat" affect, often referred to as the *negative symptoms* of schizophrenia. Some patients show both categories of symptoms, so it is not clear if there are truly different schizophrenic processes. The boundaries are quite indistinct, and there is a general lack of agreement on how the illness should be defined.

Schizophrenia seems to be reflected in some physical disorganization in the structure of certain brain regions. But we are clueless as to how they disturb the "thinking" process. Schizophrenia is a rich hunting ground for theoreticians. Yet there are reasons to seek a unifying hypothesis that would explain the common symptoms observed among sufferers of schizophrenia. The origins of the physical deficits in the schizophrenic brain are in part genetic. The lifetime probability of developing schizophrenia is about 40 percent if both parents are schizophrenic, about 15 percent if only one parent is affected, and 10 percent if a first relative suffers from schizophrenia. In identical twins the incidence of schizophrenia rises to about 50 percent, so it is not purely genetic; environmental factors must also play a role. Elevated seasonal birth rates, around the winter and spring months, suggest that such influences may play a role during development in the womb. There is also evidence that influenza during pregnancy or obstetric complications at birth can increase the incidence of schizophrenia.

Magnetic resonance imaging (MRI) is a technique that provides us with images in which brain structures may be distinguished from the fluid that bathes them. Such images have revealed that many structures associated with the temporal lobe of the cortex, such as the hippocampus and amygdala, are reduced in size in schizophrenic patients, particularly in their left hemisphere. By contrast, the *ventricles*, large reservoirs that store the fluid surrounding all brain cells, tend to be enlarged. This may be due to a slight reduction in overall brain size, such as would be expected if damage occurred early in development. Unfortunately, the magnitude of these structural abnormalities does not always correlate with the severity or progression of the illness.

Nevertheless, subtle changes in the structure and number of nerve cells in the hippocampus and prefrontal cortex are consistently reported. In the hippocampus the reduced size seems to be related to a deficit of nerve cells. The volume of the prefrontal cortex may be decreased, but, paradoxically, the number of nerve cells appears to be increased. The apparent increase in the packing of nerve cells implies that their dendrites and axons have atrophied. In other words, the meshwork of interconnections is less extensive in the prefrontal lobe of schizophrenics. This may explain the PET scan findings of altered neural activity in this brain region and also why many schizophrenics perform poorly in tests of working memory function, such as the Wisconsin card sorting task. This test requires an individual to stack cards by shape, color, and number of symbols, according to an unstated rule. After ten correct placements, the rule is changed, and the routine repeated. This task requires keeping "online" memory for previous cards and errors.

These deficits in working memory must mean that schizophrenics lack relation to, or instruction from, the outside world. For example, if thoughts occur that are not recognized as self, they could be perceived as internal voices; or if some poignant event cannot be relayed to the amygdala, an appropriate emotion cannot ensue. The eventual explanation for the symptoms of schizophrenia will not be simple.

Colorful Cures

The idea that drugs could be used to treat schizophrenia or depression was the result of pure serendipity combined with astute clinical observation. These drugs were first introduced in the mid-1950s, at which time the idea of fiddling with someone's brain chemistry was considered just short of sacrilegious. The ideas of physiologists such as Edgar Adrian, at the University of Cambridge, in England, and John Eccles, at the University of Canberra, in Australia, both Nobel prize winners, then dominated understanding of brain function. They had no need for the biochemical details of neurotransmitter function; in their view, electrical conduction along axons was all that was required to explain nerve cell communication. The emancipation of the biochemist and pharmacologist had to await a better understanding of receptor structure and the nature of neurotransmitter inactivation, for these are the prime targets of drugs that modulate brain function. But the drugs that came to dominate the treatment of depression and schizophrenia had humble origins—snake oil and coal tar.

In the middle of the nineteenth century, gas became an important source of energy. It was produced by carbonizing coal at very high temperatures, which yielded coke and coal tar as byproducts. While coke had an obvious use in blast furnaces, it took time before a use for the sticky coal-tar mess was found. Eventually, the dyes found in coal tar formed the basis for the great German dye industry and the foundation of major chemical companies, such as BASF (Badisch Anilin und Soda Fabrik). Many of these newly discovered dyes found applications in science and medicine. They could be used to stain human and animal tissues to reveal cellular and subcellular structures more clearly under the microscope. But it was Nobel Prize-winner Paul Ehrlich, a German bacteriologist and chemist, who pioneered their use in medicine. He developed the idea that infectious organisms have molecules, or "receptors," on their surfaces that are different from those on the cells of the body. He therefore reasoned that they could serve as a target for a toxic chemical that would specifically eliminate the infectious organism without harm to other cells. Since he had no method of studying colorless molecules, he made use of chemical dyes, and these provided the answer.

Thousands of dyes were screened for their antimicrobial and antiparasitic actions. Methylene blue was the first dye that Ehrlich found to be effective in treating malaria, although other dyes, such as acriflavine and suramin, eventually proved to be superior. However, methylene blue resurfaced again in France at the Rhône-Poulenc laboratories in the early 1950s. Here the chemists were investigating a series of compounds related to methylene blue, a family known as the *phenothiazines*, in the hope that they would find a better antimalarial drug. While these compounds had little effect on malaria, they were effective in blocking the action of histamine, which is involved in allergic and stress reactions. One drug they produced, promethazine, caught the attention of a French neurosurgeon named Henri Laborit. Since Laborit believed that excessive histamine could cause circulatory shock during anaesthesia, he found promethazine a useful premedication to calm and allay the fears of his patients.

Laborit was so impressed with the effects of promethazine that he asked if another, more highly sedative, compound was available. He was sent chlorpromazine, which was much more powerful as a sedative, but it was not a good histamine blocker. This drug had such remarkable tranquilizing effects on his patients that he suggested a possible use for it in the relief of agitation for those suffering from schizophrenia. Although many tried chlorpromazine for this purpose, it seemed that the doses employed were too small. But, almost independently, Jean Delay and Pierre Deniker continued to increase the dose until they found an effect. Chlorpromazine proved to be remarkably effective, not only in calming schizophrenic patients but also in diminishing their hallucinations and paranoid thoughts. In 1952 the first drug with effects on the symptoms of schizophrenia was described. By the end of the decade, over fifty million chlorpromazine (Largactil/Thorazine) prescriptions had been made out.

The second route to developing drugs effective in treating schizophrenia was, in many ways, more obvious. Ancient Hindu medicine texts had noted that extracts from the Indian snake root plant (*Rauwolfia serpentina*) were useful for several medical purposes, including the treatment of insanity. These extracts were in common use around the 1930s because Indian physicians had noted their usefulness in treating hypertension. This led chemists at the Ciba drug company to isolate an active chemical, which they called reserpine, and this drug was used to treat hypertension for many years. The background information on its use in treating insanity, the availability of a pure drug, and the success of the Delay and Deniker studies allowed the American psychiatrist Nathan Kline, then at Columbia University, to convince Ciba of the potential for using reserpine in the treatment of schizophrenia. Reserpine proved to have the same clinical effect as chlorpromazine. A second anti-schizophrenic drug had been discovered.

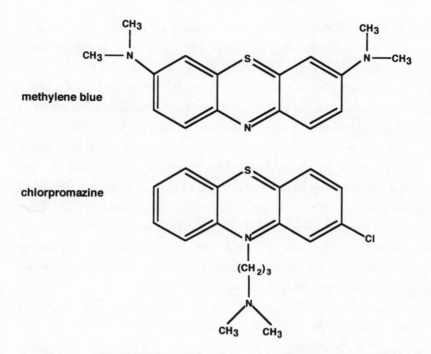

FIGURE 8.1. The similarities of chemical structure between the coal-tar dye methylene blue and the antischizophrenic drug chlorpromazine relate to the ring-like structures that are common to both.

Still no one knew how chlorpromazine or reserpine produced their remarkable effects in patients who suffered from schizophrenia; the compounds had very different structures. Yet there was one similarity. At effective concentrations both chlorpromazine and reserpine produced side effects similar to those seen in patients suffering from Parkinson's disease: a disorder of movement. About this time, techniques became available for directly measuring brain neurotransmitters, such as dopamine, serotonin, and noradrenaline. In the brains of individuals with Parkinson's disease, the dopamine content in the area that controls movement, the striatum, was found to be greatly reduced. While the administration of reserpine to rats depleted all kinds of neurotransmitters, the concomitant depletion of dopamine in the striatum was the most profound. At least in animals, the Parkinson-like effects of reserpine were explained, but its ability to relieve schizophrenia was not.

The situation was further confused during the mid-1950s, when Swedish biochemist Arvid Carlsson failed to demonstrate an effect of chlorpromazine on any transmitter in the rat brain. Yet he made one curious observation—that the levels of neurotransmitter breakdown products in the urine were significantly increased. By this time several drugs related to chlorpromazine were available and had been tested for their ability to relieve schizophrenia. When Carlsson compared their clinical efficacy with the levels of transmitter products in the urine, he found a perfect correlation for dopamine. In other words, only those drugs that increased dopamine breakdown were effective in treating schizophrenia.

This finding allowed Carlsson to propose that chlorpromazine was blocking the dopamine receptor, and that the nerve cells had increased their firing to compensate for the lack. This, he argued, resulted in an increase of transmitter turnover as well as degradation and excretion into the urine. Carlsson's theory proved to be correct when techniques developed in the mid-1970s allowed the study of how drugs bind to receptors. Chlorpromazine was demonstrated to be a dopamine antagonist. This was a crucial observation because it provided further support for the idea that schizophrenia arose from a chemical imbalance in the brain, a concept that dominated most thinking in future drug development. As both reserpine and chlorpromazine reduced the action of dopamine, the unavoidable consequence was the "dopamine hypothesis of schizophrenia": the mind had become chemically altered.

Rocket Fuel?

Given the outstanding success of chlorpromazine, chemists quickly revisited its structure in an effort to find another "miracle" drug.

The Geigy drug company found a similar compound that had languished in its basement since the late 1890s; no one had a clue what it might be useful for. A number of modifications were made to the drug, and one modified product was selected for testing and sent to the Swiss psychiatrist Roland Kuhn in the early 1950s. It had no effect. Kuhn was then sent another compound that more closely resembled chlorpromazine. It was tested on a large group of patients who had been treated previously with chlorpromazine. Many patients began to deteriorate, and their symptoms worsened. However, Kuhn noticed that the new drug tended to elevate mood in a small group of patients, an observation that led him to suggest that the drug could be useful in treating depression. The first few individuals treated for depression with the drug proved him right; he had discovered imipramine (Tofranil), the first antidepressant.

The next antidepressant to be developed had an even more remarkable origin—rocket fuel. During World War II, a mixture of liquid oxygen and ethanol was used to propel German V2 rockets. When supplies grew scarce, hydrazine was used as an alternative fuel. The copious amounts of hydrazine available after the war attracted the attention of the chemists at the Hoffmann-La Roche laboratories, who saw it as a basic building block for an array of novel chemicals for use as antibacterial agents. Using isoniazid as a starter, they produced iproniazid, which they found effective in treating tuberculosis.

Around the same time, several research groups at the Universities of Cambridge and Cardiff, in England, were investigating how the brain might eliminate neurotransmitters after they had activated their receptors. They found an enzyme, later called monoamine oxidase, that could degrade monoamine neurotransmitters, such as noradrenaline, serotonin, and dopamine. But it was Albert Zeller, a biochemist working at Northwestern University, who noted that many drugs used to treat tuberculosis, a bacterial infection that mainly affects the lungs, tended to inhibit enzymes like monoamine

oxidase, and that iproniazid was one of them. What is more, iproniazid dramatically improved the mood of tuberculosis patients and,
in laboratory rats, it dramatically reversed the Parkinson-like effects
of reserpine. All this suggested that monoamine oxidase inhibitors,
like iproniazid, might be useful in treating depression. The stage was
set for Nathan Kline, for it was he who carried out the clinical trials
that proved iproniazid to be effective in the treatment of depression.

One of the most perplexing actions of iproniazid was its ability
to reverse the Parkinson-like effects of reserpine in laboratory rats,
an outcome common to all antidepressant drugs effective in treating depression. Initially, it was suggested that iproniazid might be
some sort of "psychic energizer," but if that were so, then it was not
clear why chlorpromazine or reserpine could not have the same
effects at the right dose. Reserpine seemed, in fact, to cause depression when given to individuals to control hypertension. Many
developed severe depression and committed suicide.

Was it possible that reserpine depleted neurotransmitters other
than dopamine, and that their decrease was responsible for depression? After all, reserpine causes the depletion of all monoamine
transmitters—not only dopamine but also serotonin and noradrenaline. This was not the only problem. Imipramine, an effective
antidepressant, did not inhibit monoamine oxidase. Moreover, if
monoamine oxidase were inside the cell, in the mitochondria—
organelles responsible for respiration—it would not be available to
deactivate the released neurotransmitter. Some other mechanism
had to exist.

In the late 1950s the American neuropharmacologist Julius
Axelrod at the National Institute of Mental Health demonstrated
that the monoamine neurotransmitters, such as serotonin and
noradrenaline, are inactivated by reuptake into the nerve terminals.
He also showed that the reuptake of noradrenaline and serotonin
was blocked by imipramine, and that desipramine, another effective antidepressant, only blocked noradrenaline reuptake. Axelrod

had provided a chemical explanation for depression. This came to be known as the "monoamine hypothesis of depression," a condition associated with impaired function in the neural systems that use either noradrenaline or serotonin, or both. The monoamine hypothesis of depression was proposed in 1965, in a paper by the psychiatrist Joseph Schildkraut, which became one of the most quoted works of modern psychiatry.

The Petulant Mind

While the dizzying rate of drug discoveries in the 1950s provided treatments that had some effect in controlling the symptoms of schizophrenia and depression, no one had addressed the mood swings associated with bipolar depression. Unexpectedly, however, a treatment emerged from work in an isolated hospital in Bundoora, near Melbourne, Australia. In fact, it had been published in 1949, in a rather obscure journal to which no one had paid any attention. John Cade, an Australian psychiatrist, thought that something was overproduced in patients with mania and underproduced in depression. He must have believed that this factor would be secreted in the urine, for he started to inject the concentrated urine of psychotic individuals into the brains of guinea pigs.

Predictably, the urine was quite toxic, probably owing to the presence of uric acid. But he noted that the toxicity of urine from manic patients was always greater than that from schizophrenic or normal individuals. To further his studies, he needed to make the uric acid more soluble by converting it into a salt, which could then be dissolved in the solution used for the injection. Lithium chloride proved to be ideal for this purpose. Surprisingly, he found that lithium chloride reduced the toxicity of uric acid and produced a tranquilizing effect in animals when given alone. After a few trials on himself, he administered lithium to separate groups of patients suffering from schizophrenia, depression, and mania. The manic patients responded. John Cade had provided a basis for therapeutic intervention in mania. However, he never found the additional factor in the urine of manic individuals.

Five years later the Danish psychiatrist Mogens Schou repeated and confirmed Cade's observations on the antimanic properties of lithium. Later, in the mid-1960s, Schou made another important discovery. When lithium was given continuously to either unipolar or bipolar patients, their mood swings grew less frequent. It seemed that lithium could stabilize some system, or "switch," responsible for driving an individual into either a manic or depressed state. We still do not know the fundamental nature of this switch. But at the University of Cambridge in the mid-1980s, the English biochemist Michael Berridge provided the first glimpse of a possible mechanism that would account for such a change in synaptic function. He found that lithium blocks a cascade of events initiated by a receptor-induced enzyme, which is necessary for the transmission of the electrical impulse. Only neurons that are excessively active, such as those responsible for the mood swings accompanying mania, can be affected by lithium.

Drugs to Alter the Altered Mind

To this day the principles of drug structure and action formulated in the twenty years after the initial discoveries of the mid-1950s remain in use. Little has changed other than the chemical structure of the drugs; the basic targets at which they are directed are essentially the same. These so-called second generation drugs continue to rely on blocking serotonin and/or noradrenaline reuptake for an antidepressant action. Drugs effective in the treatment of schizophrenia are usually dopamine antagonists, although the effects of some have been attributed to an additional action at serotonin receptors. The hypotheses of dopamine overactivity as the underlying cause of schizophrenia and of serotonin/noradrenaline dysfunction as the basis of depression, and possibly mania, are still accepted today, although they remain inadequate.

The idea that monoamine oxidase inhibition was important appeared to be settled in the intervening years, although we still do not know precisely how these drugs work. There were a few problems refining these drugs for use, however. Some patients suffered liver damage with iproniazid and became jaundiced, owing to the presence of the hydrazine group in its structure. This led to the development of nonhydrazine monoamine oxidase inhibitors, such as phenelzine (Nardil) and tranylcypromine (Parnate). The monoamine oxidase inhibitors were then found to cause increased blood pressure and headache in a number of patients, which, in a few cases, led to subarachnoid haemorrhage, the rupture of a major brain blood vessel. This effect was due to tyramine, a "false" neurotransmitter found in all sorts of fermented foods, such as cheese, wine, and yogurt.

Normally, monoamine oxidase degrades tyramine in the intestine. However, when the enzyme is inhibited, as it is in individuals being treated for depression with monoamine oxidase inhibitors, tyramine gains unrestricted access to the brain. Once in the brain, tyramine activates the nerve cells that control the constriction of blood vessels, and this can lead to dangerously high blood pressure. Because tyramine is very concentrated in mature cheeses, this action has come to be known as the "cheese effect," and it led to a decline in the popularity of monoamine oxidase inhibitors—despite their effective antidepressant actions. An attempt was made to overcome the cheese effect by the development of inhibitors that only briefly block monoamine oxidase, such as moclobemide (Manerix/Aurorix) and brofaromine. But these arrived too late; drugs that inhibit the reuptake of monoamines were now perceived to be the better choice in treating depression.

The story for reuptake inhibitors is similar to that for monoamine oxidase inhibitors, although it has a happier ending. The basic structure and function of imipramine and desipramine led to the development of a whole array of drugs that were novel in structure but not in action. But a turning point in their development came with reports of decreased serotonin in the brains of suicide victims. Since many view suicide as the ultimate act of inwardly directed impulsive aggression, these reports were used to stress the havoc that could be wreaked by low levels of serotonin. Reduced levels of this simple molecule, a single neurotransmitter, soon became the biological basis for all sorts of impulsivity, depression, and suicide, as well as aggression and murder. The idea that drugs could be developed to enhance the action of serotonin and used to treat these conditions fired the imagination of researchers at the major pharmaceutical companies.

The American pharmaceutical giant Eli-Lilly heralded the era of serotonin-specific reuptake inhibitors with the introduction of Prozac (fluoxetine) in 1987. Within two years, 650,000 prescriptions of Prozac were being issued per month, and an image of its green and off-white capsule had appeared on the cover of Newsweek. Other serotonin-specific reuptake inhibitors, such as Smith Kline Beecham's paroxetine (Paxil/Seroxat), followed in the early 1990s. Other competitors' response was to produce combined serotonin and noradrenaline reuptake inhibitors, such as venlafaxine (Effexor) or mirtazepine (Remeron/Zispin), and selective noradrenaline reuptake inhibitors, such as reboxetine (Erdronax). The full cycle was complete; antidepressants now have the same actions initially reported for imipramine and desipramine but lack their unwanted effects. Moreover, this wide variety of compounds serves only to indicate that serotonin reuptake inhibition is neither necessary nor sufficient for antidepressant efficacy. All of these drugs battle for a slice of a market in which cost containment is the issue. These antidepressants would appear to have reached their apogee; it is unlikely that compounds that act on the monoamine systems will be discovered that are substantially more effective than current antidepressants. Novelty will come only when we understand the biological basis for depression. We still do not know, for example, why reuptake inhibitors specific for noradrenaline or serotonin are equally effective in the clinical management of depression.

Similarly, the development of modern antischizophrenic drugs has been based on the actions or structure of chlorpromazine, probably because reserpine was far too complex a molecule to emulate. Their action continues to be directed toward antagonizing of the various dopamine receptors. In essence, two main types of dopamine receptor exist—the D1-like dopamine receptor and the D2-like dopamine receptor. Most patients receiving these drugs show an improvement in the first few weeks of treatment irrespective of the type of dopamine receptor antagonized. Nevertheless, drugs with the greatest affinity for the D2-like dopamine receptor are clinically the most effective. Yet many investigators tend to lose sight of the fact that many of these drugs have a very high affinity for a wide variety of receptors. In the pharmacologist's parlance, they are rather "dirty" drugs, and we still do not know if their actions at other receptors are truly beneficial in the treatment of schizophrenia.

There are over a dozen antischizophrenic drugs in current use, with only about half a dozen having the same basic molecular structure. Not all phenothiazines, the chemical class to which chlorpromazine belongs, are effective antipsychotics, and not all antipsychotics are phenothiazines. A useful distinction, however, is "typical" versus "atypical," a classification that refers to the presence or absence of the unwanted Parkinson-like effects, which were originally used as an indicator of possible antischizophrenic action. Clozapine (Clozaril) was the first atypical neuroleptic. Introduced in the mid-1970s, clozapine was the first truly effective antischizophrenic drug developed since chlorpromazine. It reduced the symptoms of schizophrenia in about one-third of people who previously had not responded to the typical neuroleptics. Not only did cloza-

TABLE 8.1 Drugs Used in the Treatment of Depression

Agent	Transmitter(s) affected
Inhibitors of monoamine neurotransmitter reuptake	
Imipramine Desipramine Amitriptyline Nortriptyline Clomipramine Venlafaxine Mirtazapine[a]	Noradrenaline and serotonin
Fluoxetine Fluvoxamine Paroxetine Citalopram	Serotonin
Reboxetine	Noradrenaline
Inhibitors of monoamine neurotransmitter breakdown	
Iproniazid Phenelzine Pargyline Clorgyline Tranylcypromine Moclobemide Brofaromine	Noradrenaline and serotonin
Deprenyl[b]	Dopamine
Antimania drugs	
Lithium	Uncertain

[a] Strictly speaking, mirtazapine is not a reuptake inhibitor as its main action is believed to be the antagonism of presynaptic noradrenaline alpha-adrenoceptors, which results in increased monoamine release.

[b] Deprenyl is used mainly in the treatment of Parkinson's disease.

pine not produce the Parkinson-like effects, but it improved the negative symptoms of schizophrenia—the lack of affect or emotional response—an action not achieved by any of the drugs developed up to that time.

In comparison with earlier antipsychotic drugs, clozapine also had less of a tendency to produce the more puzzling and serious form of movement disorder known as *tardive dyskinesia*. This movement disorder, typically involving uncontrolled movements of the jaw and tongue, occurs in 20 to 40 percent of patients after months to years of antipsychotic drug treatment, and especially in those over fifty years of age. Unfortunately, clozapine was found also to suppress white blood-cell formation, a potentially lethal effect if not monitored carefully. But it served as a lead compound for the subsequent development of a range of new drugs, such as risperidone (Risperdal), olanzepine (Zyprexa), and sertindole (Serdolect), all of

---

TABLE 8.2 Dopamine Antagonists Used in the Treatment of Schizophrenia

"Typical" antagonists	"Atypical" antagonists
Chlorpromazine	Clozapine
Fluphenazine	Olanzepine
Trifluperazine	Risperidone
Thioridazine	Sertindole
Haloperidol	Remoxipride
Flupenthixol	Seroquel

The "atypical" dopamine antagonist are distinguished by their beneficial actions on both the positive and negative symptoms of schizophrenia and their lack of the unwanted movement disorders associated with the use of the "typical" antagonists. Although all drugs antagonize the action of dopamine, it must be remembered that they also affect a wide variety of other recptors.

which are effective in treating the positive symptoms of schizophrenia, and some of which have an effect on the negative symptoms.

Yet, clearly, there are limitations to the "receptor blockade" models of antidepressant and antischizophrenic drug action and design. For example, the current explanations of drug action in psychotic states do not explain the time-lag phenomenon, the delay between a drug's action at the receptor (which happens after a few hours) and its therapeutic effects (which emerge after weeks). Why one to four weeks of drug treatment is required before the depression lifts is still a mystery to most pharmacologists, although theories abound. Could it be that the continuing presence of antidepressant or antischizophrenic drugs is required to alter the activity of synapses or their pattern of connectivity in the afflicted brain circuits? Laboratory studies indicate that antidepressant treatment stimulates mechanisms required for synapse growth; and electroconvulsive therapy (ECT), an effective, if rather unpleasant, treatment for depression increases synapse numbers in parts of the temporal lobe, such as the hippocampus. On the other hand, the decreased tissue size revealed by brain imaging techniques, such as MRI scans, persists in patients following antidepressant treatment lasting three months.

It is obvious that these antischizophrenic and antidepressant drugs limit rather than control the symptoms of psychosis, a shortcoming all too evident in the treatment of schizophrenia. The clinical management of schizophrenia has been dominated by drugs that preferentially antagonize the D2-like dopamine receptor. Yet the greatest recent advance was achieved with clozapine, which has a "rich pharmacology"; in other words, it is a "dirty" drug that acts equally well at a whole variety of receptors. It is virtually impossible to pin down its precise site of action. And the action of clozapine at one or more of these receptors might account for its effectiveness in treating the negative symptoms of schizophrenia. In laboratory studies the combined action of a D2 dopamine receptor antagonist and a noradrenaline alpha-adrenoceptor antagonist results in increased dopamine activity in the prefrontal cortex. This part of the cortex is underactive in schizophrenia. Since clozapine is equally effective both as a D2-like dopamine receptor antagonist and as an alpha-noradrenaline antagonist, this dual action may serve to correct the deficiency of dopamine function in this region of the brain and thereby alleviate some of the negative symptoms of schizophrenia.

Perhaps we have focused too much on the dopamine hypothesis of schizophrenia, and other drug targets may be more effective. For example, nearly 90 percent of schizophrenics smoke. There may be many reasons for this behavior; it is possible that their illness makes them vulnerable to addiction. Alternatively, nicotine may regulate dopamine release in some yet unknown way. Or schizophrenics may benefit from its cognition-enhancing effects. It is time to take stock of the long-standing hypotheses about schizophrenia and depression, if we are to advance our quest for more effective chemical treatments.

A Unifying Hypothesis?

The English psychiatrist Tim Crow suggests that the basis for depression and schizophrenia is entirely "genetic." He argues that schizophrenia and affective disorders cannot be categorised, and that their symptoms overlap to form a continuum. Given that psychosis is universal, affecting all human populations to approximately the same degree, and that it is biologically disadvantageous, there must be some reason why it has persisted. Crow has stated that the persistence of the condition is somehow related to the development of language. That development seems to have required the two brain hemispheres to develop with a degree of independence. As a simple example, the right hemisphere can read words, but the left hemisphere is preferred if the meaning of the words, and not just their visual appearance or pattern, is to be understood.

It is proposed that the genetic event that allowed this hemispheric lateralization process to occur generated the capacity for language along with a degree of diversity in the human population that included the predisposition to psychosis. You may recall, moreover, that many of the functional abnormalities in both schizophrenia and depression appear to be localized to the left prefrontal cortex. Crow concludes that this genetic event leads back to the very origins of modern *Homo sapiens* and to that unique function that characterizes our species: the development of language. In other words, psychosis is unique to mankind; it is the cost of language. As French philosopher Michel Foucault said: "Language is the first and last structure of madness, its constituent form; on language are based all the cycles in which madness articulates its nature."

However, Crow's hypothesis fails to account for a number of observations. Stuttering or dyslexia, for example, do not necessarily lead to psychosis, and certain forms of psychosis seem to be specific to certain families. Another problem is that both schizophrenia and depression respond specifically to defined medications, which implies that different neurotransmitter systems are involved in each condition. Nevertheless, Crow's idea is very attractive. Nothing is more human than speech. Our closest primate relatives, chimpanzees, use tools, have intricate social lives, and show signs of self-awareness. But they lack spoken language and all the capacities it implies, from rapid and flexible manipulation of symbols to the ability to conceptualize things remote in time or space. Unfortunately, speech does not fossilize, although the basic brain capacity for complex language, along with the necessary mouth and throat anatomy, was probably in place before 150,000 years ago. Most of the behaviors thought to depend on language did not appear until 40,000 years ago. At that time, tools, burials, living sites, and occasional hints of art and personal adornment point to humans capable of planning and foresight, social organization and mutual assistance, a sense of aesthetics, and a grasp of symbols.

These dramatic transformations must imply one more biological change. The "fortuitous" gene mutation posited by Crow would have its origins in the evolution of human culture; it suggests a very close relationship between artistic creativity and another fundamental component of the human spirit, the religious experience—the sense of transcendence and the sacred. As English geneticist Steve Jones has put it: "Each of us is a living fossil, carrying within our genes a history that goes back to the beginning of humanity, and far beyond."

Funhouse Mirrors

The Case of the Prehistoric Doodler

So where do we seek our antecedents of the sacred—the memory of those experiential and emotional components that relate to the more thoughtful, rational components that define the human condition? And is there a pharmacological bridge to transcendence? Can chemical substances really activate latent mental mechanisms in the normal human brain and provoke ecstasy, religious experience, and a sense of cosmic, or mystical, consciousness?

The Pergouset cave in the Lot valley of southwestern France contains three chambers with fine examples of palaeolithic art, from the end of the last Ice Age, around 12,000 to 15,000 years ago. This was a time of rapid technological innovation and change that saw the development of complex social structures as hunter-gatherers evolved into the sedentary communities that came to dominate our way of life. Palaeolithic art shows evidence for organized settlements, communal graves, finely shaped tools—such as spears, hooks, burins, and scrapers—and art in the form of Venus figurines, personal ornaments, and cave paintings.

There is a fourth chamber in the Pergouset cave that can be reached only by crawling through narrow, mud-choked, steep passages. It has a sloping ceiling engraved with a fantastic bestiary, which includes long-necked creatures with monstrous heads. The sloping ceiling of the chamber makes them look almost magical or illusory; it appears as if they are emerging from the darkness of the preceding gallery or the floor below. Are these drawings the simple works of a prehistoric doodler? If so, their creator took great pains to reach this small and private niche. Perhaps they were drawings of fantasy arising from an altered state of consciousness caused by prolonged isolation, boredom, or sleep deprivation. Alternatively, the archaeologists who discovered these drawings suggest their creator could have been "stoned" on fly agaric mushroom.

Most prehistoric images were produced in full daylight, so those lying in total darkness within deep caves must have had some particular significance. Caves are secret, mysterious, and menacing places; they are totally silent, utterly dark, and completely disorientating. Upon entering a deep cave we lose many of our everyday sensory experiences and cross a boundary into an unknown world that is almost supernatural. It is easy to imagine that caves could be used for rituals, or rites of passage, to summon up supernatural forces. An obvious but simplistic extension of these ideas is that images painted on cave walls serve to reach and control supernatural forces for the benefit of their creator and his or her community. In other words, these images must be interpreted in a symbolic, rather than literal, manner. There is the story of a researcher, for example, who had identified twenty-two animal forms drawn on Australian rocks, using zoological reasoning, only to learn from a native Aborigine that he had been wrong about fifteen and only superficially right about the other seven. The art of the past no longer speaks to us in the language of its creators.

Michel Lorblanchet is a French archaeologist who specializes in studying the production of cave paintings. In one experiment he memorized a frieze that contained twenty-five animal outlines and reproduced the panel in another cave of similar dimensions, with a lamp held in his left hand. The whole exercise took him about an hour —one to four minutes for each figure. This suggests that cave painting was probably done by our ancestors in an intensive burst of creativity. He has also suggested that the creators of these cave images generated their elegant diffused haloes by holding the paint in their mouth and spit-spraying it with pursed lips in order to disperse it as fine droplets. Lorblanchet believes spit-painting may have had a symbolic significance: "Human breath, the most profound expression of a human being, literally breathes life onto a cave wall. The painter projected his being onto the rock."

But it is virtually impossible to determine if an image is symbolic. You can see the image of a horse as Pegasus (messenger of the Gods), a detail from a hunting scene, or the painter's favorite stallion. As the French sculptor Auguste Rodin put it, the creator was merely "giving shape to his dreams." The term "prehistoric art" is probably a misnomer. These images must have been a complex interweaving of the real and nonreal, the mundane and whimsical, the religious and secular. Although art is a phenomenon notoriously difficult to define, these cave images are an extension of the cultural and natural environment of their creators and are related to many aspects of human experience.

Human figures rarely exist in cave paintings; they are dominated by large animals such as bison, deer, aurochs, and horses. The human figures that do exist appear to be wearing masks, animal skins, and antlers. These may represent camouflage for hunting or a ceremonial dress worn by shamans for religious rituals involving hunting, fertility, and the initiation of the young. The term *shaman* comes from the Tungus, a Mongol tribe of central Asia, who used it to describe a person with spiritual powers. Shamans are variously described as healers, priests, magicians, and weather controllers— in essence, they were prehistory's psychotherapists. Their role was to be a liaison between their "customers" and the spirit world, a task usually requiring trances or hallucinations to attain "altered states of consciousness."

During a trance a shaman is supposed to experience *entoptics*,"
or, more properly, *phosphenes* (from the Greek *phos*, "light," and
phaino, "show"), visual phenomena that manifest as patterns of zig-
zags, chevrons, dots, grids, or vortices. These were either self-
induced by the shaman or else caused by some "magic" concoction
containing plant extracts. Entoptics, therefore, can explain the
presence of commonly encountered motifs in rock art, such as
those on the megalithic monuments at Newgrange in Ireland, as the
hallucinated forms experienced by the shaman.

Mushroom Mania

The fly agaric mushroom (*Amanita muscaria*) was used extensively
in prehistory; indeed, it continues to be used to this day. The mushroom is widespread in all temperate parts of the Northern Hemisphere, where it grows particularly well under fir and birch trees. It
is called fly agaric because of its insecticidal properties; *mukhomor*
is its traditional Russian name. The use of fly agaric is steeped in a
folklore that is whimsical but fascinating.

About 4,500 years ago Indo-Europeans moved southward into
what is now Pakistan and northern India. They settled in the Indus
Valley, where the fine fertile soil deposited by the river allowed the
development of literate urban communities. For unknown reasons
these communities collapsed, and their peoples migrated eastward
to the basin of the River Ganges, where a more lasting urban civilization was established some 3,000 years ago. Here the Aryans, who
occupied but a small part of India, composed their sacred hymns,
the Vedas.

The ninth book of the Vedas is dedicated to Soma. Soma was
identified with the moon god Chandra. However, it was Indra, the
king of gods, who popularized its use, for he was much addicted to
drinking "sweet, intoxicating Soma," quaffing some "thirty bowls at
a single draught ere he hastens to combat against hostile air

demons." The Veda contains many descriptions of Soma: it appears as a god, a juicy and fleshy red plant, juices from a plant, or the urine of a priest who had ingested the plant. The last description agrees with many modern accounts of the use of intoxicating mushrooms among the Finno-Ugrian tribes that inhabit Siberia. In these cultures the fly agaric mushroom is a prized possession. One mushroom can cost three to four reindeers, an exchange rate that is hard to believe. Moreover, it is well established that the impecunious will drink the urine of their rich kinsfolk who have consumed the mushroom because it provides even more potent effects. Depending on the "dose," this process can be effective for up to four or five times.

All of these effects are consistent with what we know of the pharmacology of *Amanita muscaria.* In the mid-1960s three separate research groups showed that the active ingredients of the mushroom are muscimol, a drug that acts as a GABA agonist, and ibotenic acid, which is the precursor to muscimol. In humans muscimol elevates body temperature and mood, causes repetition of recently experienced visual images, and induces hallucinations. But ten times the amount of ibotenic acid is needed to achieve the same effect as muscimol. This is because ibotenic acid only becomes active when it is converted into muscimol by the body. This explains the urine recycling phenomenon—or, in the language of the pharmacologist, the first-pass effect, whereby a drug becomes activated only by metabolism. It is an effect that has been used by our ancestors for thousands of years. So it is not unreasonable for Lorblanchet to assume that the prehistoric doodlings he found in the Pergouset cave were the products of an "altered vision."

From about 12,000 years ago, as the Ice Age glaciers melted, the inhabitants of Central Asia began to move into the desolate tundra and taigas, the coniferous forests lying between tundra and steppe, of the Arctic North. Later they migrated across the Bering landbridge into Arctic America. And there is little doubt that present-day Native Americans are descended from people of Asian extraction. This has been validated by evidence of numerous finds of Siberian technology, such as spear tips, that have been found in Alaska and the Yukon. Further migrations southward into new environments brought technological change, the domestication of crops and animals, and the rise of settled communities stretching as far south as Monte Verde in southern Chile. Here the inhabitants acquired an intimate knowledge of the resources available to them, including the use of medicinal plants. These migrations led ultimately to the great Maya, Inca, and Aztec empires, which were later destroyed by the descendants of their European ancestors. The links with Siberia have all but disappeared from the archaeological record. But there is at least one exception—the use of mind-altering mushrooms. For there is evidence of fly agaric use in the traditions of some Native American cultures, where it is referred to as *miskwedo*.

In Meso-America, interest centred on a mushroom termed *teonanacatl*, the "food of the gods." This seems to have been sacred, for the hundreds of mushroom stone sculptures dotted around El Salvador, Guatemala, and Mexico, dating back 2,500 years, show faces of gods or demons emerging from their stems, as if emblematic of some religious belief. Indeed, when the god-fearing conquistadors first experienced the effects of teonanacatl, its use was so ruthlessly suppressed that the properties and rituals associated with the mushroom became engulfed in secrecy. Teonanacatl was rediscovered for the West only in the mid-1950s by R. Gordon Wasson, an American banker with interest in the medicinal effects of plants, who ingratiated himself into a sacred mushroom ceremony and was allowed to return with a sample. The mushroom was found to be *Psilocybe mexicana*, and its active ingredients, psilocin and psilocybin, were isolated by the Swiss chemist Albert Hofmann in the late 1960s. But teonanacatl had another fascination for Wasson. His Russian wife, Valentina Pavlovna Wasson, like most individuals of northern Slavonic cultures, would happily gather mushrooms for consumption, whereas to him, an American of Anglo-Saxon extraction, they were repugnant, putrid, and poisonous.

To explain the rift between their two cultures, the Wassons resorted to studying the origins of peoples and their languages and came to suggest that our ancestors in the remote past had worshipped mushrooms. In some cultures the worshipful attitude survived, while in others the taboos that must have attended mushroom worship lived on in hatred and fear of all fungi. From the time early humans discovered the effects of fly agaric, probably while foraging for food, it has been the focus of Siberian shamanism. The mushroom grew in association with the birch, and this became the "Tree of Life" in Siberian folklore. The Wassons argued, therefore, that this mushroom cult spread from Siberia, in prehistory, to form the basis of modern religion. In the Garden of Eden, as in Siberia, the serpent was the spirit of the Tree of Life. Similarly, in Meso-America, the Aztecs revered another plant, a cactus, which they referred to as *peyotl*. This cactus became a key element in the religious ceremonies of the Mexican Indians, who resisted its suppression by the conquistadors by integrating its use into the Christian beliefs of their conquerors; peyotl use persists to this day as one of the "sacraments" in the religion of these Mexican Indians.

Peyotl is a beautiful green cactus (*Lophophora williamsii*) crowned with tufts of silky hairs. Its active ingredient is mescaline. The German chemist Arthur Heffter isolated mescaline in 1896 and consumed various amounts of the extract in order to confirm its psychoactive properties. But it was English novelist Aldous Huxley who popularized mescaline by publishing his personal experiences of the drug in his book *The Doors of Perception* (1954). Because mescaline is a fairly weak drug, those who use peyotl say that it in no way resembles eating the cactus, which probably contains many more psychoactive substances. Many researchers have modified the basic structure of mescaline to obtain more potent drugs.

Mescaline, however, does not have to be the basic building block; others are more readily available. Elemicin, for example, the starting material for trimethoxyamphetamine (TMA), is present in the oil of nutmeg (*Myristica fragrans*). Before his conversion to Islam, the imprisoned American civil rights activist Malcolm X used nutmeg when his supplies of marijuana ran out. The preparation of methylenedioxymethylamphetamine (MDMA), or ecstasy, can be started using safrole, which is abundantly present in sassafras oil. It was the chemist Alexander Shulgin who first synthesised TMA in the mid-1960s, when working at the Dow chemical company. Since then he has synthesized and tested a whole array of these so-called phenethylamines, which he has meticulously recorded in a book called *PIHKAL* (Phenethylamines I Have Known And Loved), written with his wife Ann Shulgin. It is essential reading for all forensic chemists who are hard pressed to keep up with the innovations of their colleagues in underground laboratories.

Acid Metaphysics

You may recall from earlier mention that *kykeon*, that elusive brew of the ancient Greeks, is believed to have been prepared from a fungus-infected barley (*Claviceps purpurea*). The fungus that has infected the barley is generally referred to as ergot, and the chemicals it produces are quite toxic. They cause narrowing of the blood vessels (vasoconstriction) and can lead to brain seizures and gangrene of the limbs due to reduced blood supply. This condition is called ergotism and, in the Middle Ages, was referred to as St. Anthony's Fire, because the blackened gangrenous limbs and burning sensations were believed to be the retribution for sin, and sufferers invoked St. Anthony, who could protect against fire, infection, and epilepsy. Yet this toxic fungus was also used to aid childbirth because the muscle contractions it produced facilitated delivery and reduced subsequent bleeding.

This folklore attracted the attention of chemists at the Sandoz pharmaceutical company who isolated ergotamine and ergonovine from the *Claviceps* fungus in the early 1900s. As expected, these compounds were found to contract blood vessels, and they are still used in the treatment of migraine, which is due, in part, to a dilatation of blood vessels. The chemists used the common structure of these drugs to prepare an array of compounds in the hope that one or more would find a clinical use. Albert Hofmann was the chemist committed to synthesizing the twenty-fifth compound in the series. In the final stages, which involved crystallization, he was overcome with unusual sensations characterized by "an extremely stimulated imagination." He had probably absorbed some of the compound through his skin, since, in those days, safety regulations were a little more lax and the use of protective gloves was uncommon.

Returning to the laboratory, Hofmann decided to try ingesting 250 micrograms, a dose we now know to be about two and a half times that needed to achieve the drug's hallucinogenic effects. He recalled his experiences as follows: "My field of vision wavered and was distorted. . . . Pieces of furniture assumed grotesque, threatening forms. . . . The lady next door a malevolent, insidious witch with a colored mask. . . . A demon had invaded me, had taken possession of my body, mind, and soul." Hofmann had discovered LSD (lysergic acid diethylamide), the most potent psychedelic drug known to humankind. Bedlam followed.

In the early 1960s LSD left the research laboratory. John Beresford, who had been involved in LSD research, purchased a gram of Delysid (LSD) from Sandoz and Michael Hollingshead, author of *The Man Who Turned On the World,* ended up with some of this diluted in sugar in a mayonnaise jar. One of the people he "turned on" with a sample was Timothy Leary, a Harvard University lecturer in psychology who was researching the effects of psilocybin. Leary was so impressed with LSD that he placed an order with Sandoz for a hundred grams, no less than about a million doses!

Together with his colleagues Richard Alpert and Ralph Metzner, they started to investigate the effects of LSD. The Harvard administration became uneasy as these intrepid investigators used the experimental drugs themselves along with their research subjects. The party-like atmosphere brought ridicule from other researchers who wanted to know how scientific objectivity could be maintained if the investigators were also using mind-altering drugs.

Leary's students introduced the drug, as LSD-laced sugar cubes, to the coffee shops and clubs surrounding Harvard. Its use spread to the West Coast, where cliques partied with "electric Kool-Aid," an LSD-laced punch, to the rock-and-roll music of The Grateful Dead. LSD had taken off. Hollywood glamorized it; Cary Grant was using LSD as some form of psychotherapy. The American Beat writers Jack Kerouac and Ken Kesey, and poet Allen Ginsberg were using LSD for metaphysical purposes. The U.S. Army wanted Hofmann to synthesize kilograms of the drug for chemical warfare. The Central Intelligence Agency was testing LSD on unwitting subjects.

Sober society was becoming anxious about the enormous popularity of LSD. Many "insane hippies" were killing themselves during mind-altering "trips"; the drug was linked to the crazed killing of American actress Sharon Tate by the murderous Charles Manson gang. There was a climate of dissent; the fabric of society was viewed as under threat. LSD had become associated with the perceived "good" of Eastern mysticism. America was at war with a largely Buddhist nation, and the war was opposed vehemently by these "hippies."

The response of the government was sharp. Leary was arrested and given a thirty-year sentence for possession of cannabis. LSD was alleged to cause chromosome damage and labeled a second thalidomide. Finally, in 1971, the United Nations Convention on Psychotropic Substances extended international drug control to include LSD in Schedule I, the most restrictive class of substances with no medical value. The LSD era was all but over except for continued underground production to supply a small but lasting demand. A medical use for LSD was never found. Like ecstasy today, LSD was the fashion of an era.

Getting High

The effects of LSD cannot be defined in absolute terms; we have only the subjective reports of users. In many ways the experiences described often reflect the individual's personal expectations of what the drug is likely to do for them. If the user wishes to acquire a sense of the "inner self," then it is likely that the sensations experienced will range from deep religious feelings to a discernment of self-awareness. The hope that LSD will provide a "mind-blowing" experience might explain why some users believe they can fly and so jump out of windows to prove the point.

Reports of altered perception are usually visual and involve extreme distortion of the physical environment and specific objects. One of the most fascinating and frequent effects of LSD is transmutation of the senses. This is referred to as *synesthesia*, an example being the perception of sounds as colors. As with all psychoactive drugs, when an individual takes LSD in poor mood or dismal surroundings, it can produce terrifying experiences, including the of loss of control and an inability to return to normality. He or she may literally become paralyzed with fear. These experiences are often referred to as a having a "bad trip."

A single 100-microgram dose of LSD is usually enough to produce significant effects that last from six to twelve hours. But one can "sense something" with as little as 25 micrograms. When LSD is taken frequently, tolerance quickly builds up. But this tolerance is rapidly lost, within three to four days of abstinence, and without any withdrawal symptoms. LSD does not appear to be an addictive drug. Animals have no taste for it and fail to self-administer the drug repeatedly when given the opportunity to do so. One common unwanted effect, however, is "flashbacks," usually in the form of altered visual perceptions weeks to months after the drug has been used. Since the drug is rapidly eliminated from the body, these cannot be a direct effect of LSD but are probably caused by some related action, which may unmask existing emotional problems (they are more common in people who tend to fantasize).

Because hallucinations are a common symptom of schizophrenia, many researchers have suggested that LSD may provide some understanding of this illness. However, it is quite misleading to compare the hallucinations experienced in schizophrenia to the altered perceptions induced by LSD. In schizophrenia the most common form of hallucination is auditory, a specific voice, clearly distinct from that of the patient, which speaks in sentences or fragments of sentences. Hallucinations in the schizophrenic are lifelong, whereas the visual illusions induced by LSD occur only when the drug is present, except in the small minority of individuals who experience flashbacks. What is more, schizophrenics in remission say that LSD-induced reactions are very different from those they experience in their psychotic periods, and psychiatrists have little difficulty in discriminating between drug-induced effects and the symptoms of schizophrenia. "Genuine" hallucinations are characterized by perceptions that are superimposed on the environment, such as the visual distortion of objects, and that are usually threatening, such as the perception of individuals as malevolent. For these reasons, psychiatrists Humphrey Osmond and Abram Hoffer introduced the term *psychedelic* in 1954 to refer to substances that in small doses can alter perception, thought, and mood to create illusions in the mind of the user. So LSD is more correctly a psychedelic rather than a hallucinogen.

Sorting out how psychedelic drugs work has not been a straightforward task, and their precise action still remains unclear. Drugs such as LSD, psilocybin, or mescaline bear a structural resemblance to the brain neurotransmitters noradrenaline and serotonin, which regulate our state of arousal and mood. The raphe nucleus of the brain stem, which sends axons using the serotonin neurotransmitter to many brain regions, is involved in psychedelic drug action. If rats are given LSD or psilocybin, the cells of the raphe nucleus cease to fire—an interesting observation since this region of the brain regulates the dreaming phases of sleep.

Given that LSD binds to serotonin receptors, a common belief is that it reduces the release of serotonin from the presynapse, which would explain why nerve cells cease to fire in the raphe nucleus. So psychedelic drugs could induce the intense emotions and vivid imagery of the dream state while the subject is awake. Unfortunately, there are problems with this convenient idea. Mescaline, for example, does not have this effect, and some nonpsychedelic drugs related to LSD readily inhibit firing in the raphe nucleus. Indeed LSD given to drug-tolerant individuals can silence the raphe cells, despite their inability to experience its psychedelic actions. Clearly, other mechanisms in different brain regions must be involved.

The locus coeruleus in the brain stem lies beside the raphe nucleus and also sends axons to many brain regions; these, unlike the raphe cells, use noradrenaline as their neurotransmitter. If the locus coeruleus is electrically stimulated, it produces a dramatic behavioral response in rats: they become hyper-responsive to all forms of stimuli in the environment. They are easily startled, jumping if a novel sound is suddenly presented, or they tend to stare as if in a state of panic. Although it is difficult to infer what a rat may be feeling, their reaction is similar to the intense response to external stimuli observed in individuals under the influence of a psychedelic drug. Furthermore, the response is different from the behavioral activation of this brain region that is produced by amphetamines.

There is another important difference: psychedelic drugs increase the firing rate of the locus coeruleus, whereas amphetamines do not. It was therefore quite surprising to find that direct injection of psychedelic drugs into the locus coeruleus had no effect on the firing rate. Obviously, the drugs were affecting some region of the brain that serves as a regulator of the locus coeruleus. We are still unclear about the circuitry involved, but it must at least involve both the locus coeruleus and the raphe nucleus. These areas are sometimes collectively referred to as the *reticular activating system*, because their individual contributions maintain our state of consciousness, such as our ability to sleep or to be aroused.

The effects of psychedelic drugs on the reticular activating system may provide a clue to how they work. Activation of the locus coeruleus by psychedelic drugs results in a patterned release of noradrenaline throughout the brain and a powerful alerting action that is much more profound than that achieved with amphetamines. This state of profound arousal may impair the ability to compare and contrast sensory stimuli that are otherwise perceived normally and interrelated coherently. Instead they may become chaotic; sounds may be perceived as colors. Such extremely enhanced states of alertness may also account for the intensity that psychedelic drugs confer on our perception of sensory stimuli.

However, it is hard to believe that psychedelic drugs confer on us a sense of "inner self"—the "transcendent" state so often eulogized by writers such as Aldous Huxley, Timothy Leary, and many others. If this view of their mode of action is in any way correct, one cannot begin to imagine how psychedelic drugs can reveal our sense of divinity, let alone the cardinal reason for being human. The problem with this thinking is that it always has a whiff of the Orient, like that associated with the smoking of opium. After all, LSD is a thoroughly Western drug; Hofmann made it in Switzerland.

Quixotic Potions

Humankind's preoccupation with psychedelic drugs is a basic feature of all the arcana exhumed from our past—from the ergot grain goddesses of Greece to the peyotl cults of Mexico. Only a few of these psychedelic substances have been considered in any depth. Many more exist, and they all can influence brain pathways that use either serotonin or noradrenaline, since most contain compounds closely related to LSD, although not as potent. *Ololiuqui*, an Aztec brew made from the seeds of *Rivea corymbosa* contains lysergic acid amide, sometimes referred to as ergine. And there is the *ayahuasca* potion of South America. It is prepared from the climbing plant *Banisteriopsis caapi*, a liana, although it usually contains a mixture of plant ingredients made to the shaman's individual recipe. Harmine, a chemical substance that prevents the breakdown of neurotransmitters such as noradrenaline and serotonin, is the principal ingredient of the liana, but it is unlikely to provide the psychedelic effects of ayahuasca. Harmine probably prevents the breakdown of dimethyltryptamine, a compound that is related to psilocybin and which is found in some of the plants added to the ayahuasca. In fact, dimethyltryptamine is found in many other plants used for their "mind-altering properties." Examples include the "psychedelic snuffs" known as *cohoba*, made from the plant *Mimosa hostilis*, or *yopo*, from *Anadenanthera peregrina*, which are blown up the nose using tubes specially designed for that purpose.

TABLE 9.1 Neurotransmitter Systems Influenced by Psychedelic Drugs

Agent	Transmitter(s) affected
Muscimol	GABA agonist
Lysergic acid diethylamide Psilocin Psilocybin Mescaline Dimethyltryptamine	Serotonin agonists/antagonists?

Not all psychedelic experiences are caused by chemicals that resemble LSD, psilocybin, or mescaline. For example, the active ingredient of fly agaric is muscimol, which activates the GABA receptor. We still do not know how this action creates a psychedelic experience—like LSD, it may inhibit the release of serotonin. Another example is the use of drugs that block the action of the acetylcholine neurotransmitter. The alleged "flying ointments" of witches in medieval Europe were oil extracts of black henbane (*Hyoscyamus niger*), deadly nightshade (*Atropa belladonna*), and mandrake (*Mandragora officinarum*), all of which contained a mixture of the acetylcholine antagonists atropine, hyoscine, and scopolamine. This mixture is deadly, since large doses result in cardiac arrest and respiratory collapse. These unwanted effects can be circumvented to some degree if the salve is applied to areas of the skin enriched with blood vessels, such as the armpit, rectum, or vagina. Hence the image of the witch who flies on the "greased shaft" of the broomstick. Recently, some intrepid individuals have prepared these salves according to the ancient "recipes" and, after liberal application to the skin, fell into a deep sleep and experienced sensations of flying. There is no reason to doubt their report; these awful concoctions are probably able to produce all sorts of bizarre effects.

Artificial Paradise

Whether called hashish, kef, charas, bhang, ganja, marijuana, or, in scientific circles, the flowering tops of the female hemp plant (*Cannabis sativa*), the very words used to describe cannabis carry romantic overtones. Scarcely seen in Europe until the middle of the nineteenth century, cannabis was known only by reputation from the tales of travelers returning from the Orient. It was familiar to the Chinese Emperor Shen Nung, whose work on pharmacy was written almost 5,000 years ago. And 2,500 years ago, the Greek writer Herodotus described mysterious Scythian hordes, who would throw cannabis on hot rocks in their sweat lodges and become inebriated by inhaling the vapors. The delights of cannabis have been recounted in the colourful tales of Scheherazade in *The One Thousand and One Nights*, and by Marco Polo, who told of Hassan-ben-Sabbah and how he used cannabis to seduce young men into war against the Infidel—the sect of the Hachichins, from which the modern word assassin derives.

Cannabis reached France with the return of Napoleon's soldiers from Egypt, but in Paris cannabis became glorified by members of Le Club des Hachichins, such as Théophile Gautier and Charles Baudelaire. Central to this group of notorious writers was Jacques-Joseph Moreau (de Tours), for it was he who provided the cannabis. But unlike Baudelaire and Gautier, who used cannabis to enliven their writings, Moreau's interests were more scientific. He had observed the intoxicating effects of cannabis in Algeria, where it is served as a confection called *dawamesc*. This is prepared by grinding the hemp tops together with sugar, orange juice, cinnamom, cloves, cardamon, nutmeg, musk, pistachios, and pine kernels; the mixture is served in portions no bigger than the size of a hazel nut. It was dawamesc that Moreau purveyed to Le Club des Hachichins.

The loosening of associations, clouding of consciousness, personality changes, and perceptual distortions induced by cannabis were meticulously recorded by Moreau, because he believed that these semipsychotic states might have implications for our understanding of mental illness, a daring idea in nineteenth-century France. However, in *Les Paradis artificiels*, published in 1860, Baudelaire was careful to explain that the "hallucinations" induced by hashish were not true hallucinations. The hallucination is progressive, almost voluntary, and ripens only through the action of the imagination. In the view of Baudelaire, who was a careful observer, unlike Gautier, and not given to hyperbole, "Hashish will be for man's [*sic*] familiar thoughts and impressions a mirror that exaggerates but always a mirror."

Cannabis can be consumed in a number of ways; marijuana, a crude mixture of dried and crumbled leaves, small stems, and flowering tops, is the most familiar form. This is usually rolled and smoked as a cigarette, but it may also be baked into small cakes and eaten. The potency of marijuana can also depend on plant variety and method of cultivation. One method is to prevent pollination and, as a consequence, seed production in the female plant. Marijuana produced by this method is called sinsemilla (meaning "without seeds"). Hashish is another form of cannabis. This is the resinous exudate of the plant, and it contains a high concentration of cannabinoids. This resinous material is compacted into a hard, brownish mass, and small quantities are crumbled into tobacco and smoked. An extract of hashish, termed "cannabis oil," is the purest form of the drug; it, too, is added to tobacco for smoking.

Not surprisingly, cannabis influences the brain in a manner that is completely different from all the other psychedelic drugs described thus far. There are over sixty psychoactive chemicals in cannabis, collectively referred to as cannabinoids, but one called tetrahydrocannabinol is believed to be the most potent constituent. Tetrahydrocannabinol blocks, or antagonizes, the actions mediated by a specific brain receptor called the *cannabinoid receptor*. This receptor normally uses a neurotransmitter (which due to its fat-like nature is unique), called *anandamide*, the Sanskrit word for "bliss." Cannabinoid receptors are especially prevalent in those brain regions involved in regulating memory formation, such as the hippocampus. In this region of the brain, cannabis may block the release of the acetylcholine neurotransmitter, which plays an important role in learning and memory.

This may explain why cannabis use results in difficulties with problem solving and tasks that require the use of logic. But we still cannot explain the mechanism that accounts for the subjective and behavioral effects commonly associated with marijuana intoxication—feelings of euphoria and exhilaration, talkativeness and laughter, increased hunger and thirst. And, as with all psychoactive drugs, context, personality, previous experiences, and expectations play a role in the eventual consequences of cannabis use. Users can feel calm and relaxed or restless and agitated.

The most controversial claim about cannabis is that it can produce an "amotivational state." But this is not an official diagnosis— it is used to describe young people who lack goal-directed activities, and when cannabis use accompanies these symptoms, the drug is often cited as the cause. There is no evidence that cannabis damages brain cells or produces any permanent functional change in the brain. A few doses of cannabis will produce a tolerance to its effects, but this disappears rapidly and without any obvious withdrawal symptoms. Yet cannabis remains a restricted substance, no doubt due to the purges of Harry Anslinger, a commissioner of the United States Federal Bureau of Narcotics, in the 1930s.

The Pharmacology of the Infinite

Therapeutic Nihilism

Anyone dredging through the pharmacy of our prehistory would quickly recognize that many of the substances in this ancient *materia medica* could only have been inert. The Ebers Papyrus of Ancient Egypt documents 842 prescriptions and mentions more than 700 drugs, including fly specks scraped from the wall, the blood of eunuchs, grated human skull, and, above all, dung—especially crocodile dung. Perhaps this should not be so surprising: after all, for prehistoric humankind drug therapy cannot have been the first option for treating disease, since sickness came upon them in frightening and mysterious ways. Being imaginative and rational, they must have concluded that supernatural countermeasures were required. The magic thus invoked must have ultimately been reinforced by customs that used plants or other substances that brought friendly spirits to counter the evil powers of the disease. Illness was a divine punishment, and healing a purification, or catharsis, of the evil power or spirit.

This idea of catharsis is still maintained in religious ideology, as in the ultimate sacrifice of Jesus Christ who gave his life to purify the sins of humankind. Indeed, in the Middle Ages, Christ was often referred to as the Apothecary of the Soul. Most religions have well-known holy places where miraculous cures are promised. Even the father of psychoanalysis, Dr. Sigmund Freud, admitted, "I do not think our cures can compete with those of Lourdes." More secular examples abound. The "laying on of hands" is one of the oldest and most persistent treatments: the royal touch for scrofula or other skin disorders; or that of Valentine Greatrakes, seventeenth-century English Puritan soldier and merchant, for the ague and many other conditions. The work of psychiatrists in externalizing or verbalizing the forbidden impulses of their patients is, perhaps, another example.

Taken in this context, the filth of the excrements in the medicaments of prehistory must have been used to repel evil spirits of the body. Even Robert Boyle, the British founding father of modern chemistry, in 1692, was happy to recommend potions containing worms, horse dung, human urine, and moss from a dead man's skull. After all, the clay tablets and papyri that have survived the passage of time are only partly legible and are probably only a small part, a "few pages," of a longer document that may have included aspects of the spiritual, such as incantations and supplications. Clearly, magic and empiricism each played an important role in finding and employing remedies. Catharsis was at first spiritual and later pharmacological.

However, the presumed perspicacity of our ancient healers contains much that is glamorized, sentimentalized, and exaggerated because almost nothing is known about the effectiveness of their drugs. It was only occasionally, and at great intervals, that anything really serviceable was introduced into medical practice. The first truly effective medication was the introduction in 1638 of the quinine-containing Jesuit's bark (*Cinchona*), which is specific for the treatment of malaria and no other fevers. And British Navy physicians, such as John Lind, aboard the *Salisbury* in 1747, had noted the use of fresh citrus fruits for the treatment of scurvy. Was pharmacy's prehistory nothing other than a series of placebos—treatments used to alleviate a disease but in actual fact ineffective for the condition?

George Bernard Shaw has the essence of placebo in his description of Dr. Sir Ralph Bloomfield Bonnington, a character in his play *The Doctor's Dilemma*: "Cheering, reassuring, healing by the mere incompatibility of disease or anxiety with his welcome presence. Even broken bones, it is said, have been known to unite at the sound of his voice." But it was American Harry Beecher who made the idea of the placebo effect respectable. As a surgical anaesthetist during World War II, he preferred the use of morphine because it reduced the risk of cardiovascular shock. As supplies ran low, he observed on many occasions that a saline injection prevented the cardiovascular shock. In some way the saline, or placebo, appeared to be an important treatment in its own right. Convinced of the effect, he returned to Harvard and continued to study the placebo response during the mid-1950s. The placebo effect is especially important in psychopharmacology.

Nowadays, to ensure that new drugs have therapeutic value, they are tested in patients assigned randomly to groups that receive either the drug or a placebo, usually a simple sugar pill. Neither patient nor doctor knows how they were distributed until the trial is complete. This procedure is known as the *double-blind randomized placebo-controlled trial*. In the development of drugs to treat conditions of pain, anxiety, or depression, all of which have a strong psychological component, patients receiving the placebo often respond well. It is not uncommon for 65 percent of patients who receive an antidepressant drug to show signs of improvement, but up to 35 percent of patients receiving the placebo also improve. All sorts of reasoning have been invoked to explain this phenomenon. Taking part in the trial and the accompanying attention may have a positive effect on the patient; the participants may have varying degrees of depression; or the placebo may be identified because it lacks typical unwanted effects known to the patient (for example, some antidepressants cause drying of the mouth).

These significant placebo effects tend to suggest that the modern drugs that are developed for schizophrenia and depression are less effective than those previously used. Yet this cannot be the case, because older drugs were identified without using the double-blind randomized placebo-controlled trial. Is this why the legions of researchers throughout the world cannot come up with something new and more effective? For such a reliable phenomenon, which has such major implications for the development of new and more efficacious therapies for mental illness, it is remarkable that the placebo effect has not attracted scientific attention. In the meantime, in the United States alone, the Food and Drug Administration estimates that $30–40 billion are spent annually on unproven medications and vitamin supplements for health. This does not include money and time spent on psychic healing and the fads of excessive jogging and communing with nature to destroy malignant cells. The fact that placebos elude a ready explanation tells us how far we are from creating a science complex and subtle enough to encompass the human mind. The philosopher Michel Foucault talks about modern ideas not as being "correct," but as ideas of "an era from which we have not yet emerged."

Placebo and pharmacy have coexisted since the beginning of recorded time, and only in our own century have they been gradually placed into separate categories. Wherever civilization arises, we find pharmacy, because it fulfils one of the basic needs of humankind. The interesting accounts of premodern pharmacy and its rich *materia medica* can only be read to a certain extent in Western languages, because the linguistic challenges and dating of ancient evidence are so often speculative. Ruins in the river valleys of the Nile, Tigris, and Euphrates must once have throbbed with magnificent civilizations as remarkable in their own time as the later, more westernly cultures that they helped to shape. This is where the pharmacy of the West has its early antecedents, but many centuries were to pass before we had a new interpretation of the causes of disease.

The Death of Dioscorides

In the aftermath of the victorious sweep of Alexander the Great through the Eastern world, the Greek way of thought spread over an enormous area. The founding of Alexandria soon overshadowed the importance of Athens, the old seat of Greek wisdom. Around 2,400 years ago, a school of medical thought developed in Alexandria, where a sect called the Empiricists followed the teachings of Hippocrates. According to this system, the body contained four humors: blood, which was hot and moist, came from the heart; phlegm, which was cold and moist, came from the brain; yellow bile, which was hot and dry, came from the liver; and black bile, which was cold and dry, came from the spleen and bowel. In this theory the correct balance of the four humors was essential for health, and any disturbance in this balance led to disease.

Before, during, and after the time of the Greek physician Hippocrates, there was another group of botanists called the *rhizotomoi*, who became established as experts in the collection and sale of medicinal plants. Their plant drawings formed the basis for the Greek physician Dioscorides' classic treatise *De materia medica libri quinque*, which was written around 2,000 years ago. This was translated into English in 1665 and is still kept in print. It represents an intellectual milestone in the development of pharmacy, for it was written in the spirit of applied science. Dioscorides not only described the drugs of his time and explained their effects but also arranged his descriptions systematically.

In the second century A.D. the Greek physician Galen proposed that medicaments could alleviate imbalance of the humors in disease and restore the individual to health. Of particular importance was his attempt to classify the medicaments he used according to the response of the humors, rating their ability to counteract specific diseases on a scale of four degrees. Drugs with only one quality were classified as simples, whereas those with more qualities were classed as composites. Galen prepared these medicaments personally and had a very high opinion of their efficacy. There were more than 470 drugs of vegetable, animal, and mineral origin, and a profusion of medical formulae in his armamentarium. Galen's ideas persisted for 1,500 years, owing to the sheer logic of his system and a reverence for his authority.

Following the demise of Greco-Roman culture, Arabic manuscripts assumed an important significance to the pharmacy of the Western world, from the ninth to thirteenth centuries. Of these, the work of the Persian physician Avicenna was of considerable influence, since one text contained descriptions of more than 700 drugs, and another, more specialized text described drugs that specifically affected the heart. The armamentarium became considerably enlarged, because Persian and Indian drugs were unknown to the Greco-Roman world. Pharmacy emerged as the art of knowing *materia medica* and preparing compounded medications as prescribed and ordered by the physician. The pharmacist became readily distinguishable from the alchemist and physician. Sicily and Spain played an important role in channeling this Greco-Arabic medicine into the West in the seventh to twelfth centuries. Sicily was a center of Arabic culture, and cities in Spain, such as Toledo, served in the translation of Arabic texts for Western scholars.

During the early Middle Ages, as the Germanic tribes swept through Europe, fortified by the belief that healing powers lay with the gods and not with science, the manuscripts of pharmacy became exclusively restricted to the clergy, hidden away in their safe asylums of learning. Thus was born monastic medicine, dogmatic and with the added important component of faith. However, Arabic influence continued to increase in the famous eighth-century school at

Salerno, which attracted not only patients but also students. In the eleventh century, public pharmacies began to appear, initially in southern Italy and France. Between 1231 and 1240, the German Emperor Frederick II issued an edict that became a legal milestone and heralded the profession of pharmacy. It separated the pharmaceutical profession from the medical profession, required official supervision of pharmaceutical practice, and obliged the taking of an oath to prepare drugs reliably in a uniform and of suitable quality.

This marked the start of the Renaissance, during which experimental methods were developed that eventually revealed fallacies in the brilliant writings of Galen and laid the concept of humors to rest. And with the Renaissance came Paracelsus. Paracelsus was the Swiss physician whose name was originally Theophrastus Bombastus von Hohenheim, a sixteenth-century philosopher, chemist, and physician, who introduced the concept of the body as a chemical laboratory and the use of chemical remedies as a matter of principle and study. The definition of chemical drugs was created. While many would come to the same conclusions later, he should not be considered to be too "modern," for he still believed that the heavenly bodies influenced the organs of the body and the remedies used against disease.

But François de le Boë Sylvius founded the true medico-chemical doctrine in the seventeenth century. It was a hybrid of ideas taken from Galen and Paracelsus. He believed that food was transformed by the saliva and fermented by secretions from the pancreas. This resulted in either acid or alkaline products; when both were in balance the person was deemed healthy, but when in imbalance disease resulted. The theory became a basis for preparing new chemical drugs. Combined with the arrival of new drugs from the Americas, such as *Cinchona* bark, the idea of drug specificity further undermined the old Galenic ideas and the belief that the books of Dioscorides and Avicenna contained all of the drug lore in the world.

In the eighteenth century progress remained slow, because physicians lacked the experimental techniques for establishing the site and the mechanism of drug action. This all changed with the arrival of the German pathologist Rudolf Virchow in the nineteenth century. Virchow founded cellular pathology. In his view, "the organism is not unified but a social arrangement"; the cell was the bearer of life and disease the reaction of the cell to abnormal stimulation, a theory that was seminal to the later drug-development work of Paul Ehrlich, the German biochemist Gerhard Domagk, and British bacteriologist Alexander Fleming. As Virchow was formulating his ideas on cellular pathology, François Magendie, in France, began to repudiate any scientific opinion that could not be supported by observation or experimental findings, believing that drugs could be given to humans only if their effectiveness had been first demonstrated in animals. His student, Claude Bernard, was more closely aligned to establishing the principles of drug action—how they were absorbed, distributed in the body, and eliminated by metabolism. In the late nineteenth century Oswald Schmiedeberg advanced the work of Bernard. Not only was he a good chemist, but he also used the drugs to demonstrate their effects on animals and organ preparations, procedures now commonly used in all research laboratories. In 1872 Schmiedeberg assumed the chair of pharmacology at the newly founded Imperial University at Strasbourg, France. Here he established a model institute in which he created the subject of pharmacology as we know it today.

One notable achievement of researchers at the Strasbourg institute was the first isolation of pure deoxyribonucleic acid—a component of nuclein that had been isolated from pus cells by the Swiss biochemist Johann Friedrich Miescher in Tübingen, Germany, in 1869. Deoxyribonucleic acid is the basic unit of our DNA, through which we transfer all of our genetic information. The chemical and physical nature of DNA was elucidated by scientists, such as Erwin Chargaff, Max Delbrück, Rosalind Franklin, Linus Pauling,

Alexander Todd, and Maurice Wilkins—information that allowed James Watson and Francis Crick to formulate their conception of DNA as a double helix in 1953. This was one of the most significant discoveries of the twentieth century, and it ushered in modern molecular biology, the milieu in which research is conducted today.

Drug Driven

Drug Symbiosis

Genetic information is present in every cell of our body in the form of chromosomes. There are a total of forty-six chromosomes—twenty-three pairs—in each human cell. The main constituent of chromosomes is DNA. This long thread is composed of relatively small molecules, called *nucleotides*, and their sequence carries our genetic information. The DNA thread is most probably continuous within the chromosome, and its great length is due to the average number of nucleotides—over 100 million—contained there. In spite of the apparent continuity, one can recognize shorter segments in the DNA that have specific functions, and these are called *genes*. A chromosome may contain, on average, many thousands of genes, each made up of thousands more nucleotides. Collectively, genes are referred to as the *genome*.

The genes contained in our chromosomes are copied, almost without error, when cells divide. If, however, a gene-copying error occurs, it is called a *mutation*. Mutations can arise by the addition, deletion, or incorrect placement of one or more nucleotides. In some cases an entire gene can be duplicated or deleted. Mutation may have trivial or serious consequences, depending on how the protein encoded by the gene is altered in structure. This is because the readout from gene to protein often determines protein shape and as a consequence, the ability of the protein to function properly. Alternative forms of a gene are called *alleles.*

Allelic differences are not transmitted to descendants unless they are present in the germ cells—either sperm or egg. The union of a sperm and egg generates a new cell, which has twenty-three pairs of chromosomes, each of which contains a maternal and a paternal chromosome. Further divisions of this cell generate the embryo, which will eventually lead to the birth of an individual who carries the new allele. If the first individual carrying the allele reaches adulthood and has several offspring, there is a high chance that it will be found in later generations and become more and more frequent in succeeding generations. This is the elementary process of natural selection—Darwin's proposed model of evolution.

Since a specific allele rarely recurs in other individuals, its fate depends on natural selection and the migration of populations carrying the allele. Natural selection is the automatic choice for the stronger type, and it can make an initially rare allele the most common in a population, providing that it is advantageous to the individuals that carry it. Alleles, therefore, are clumsy but wonderful biological adaptations. They arise by trial and error, in a historical process, when they offer acceptable solutions to the needs of the species. But they inevitably set later constraints on the evolutionary process, because the DNA sequence that makes an allele different is not reversible.

Certain alleles can alter the sensitivity of some human populations to the effects of certain drugs. Sensitivity to the effects of alcohol is one of the best-studied examples. When alcohol is metabolized in the body, it is first broken down to a chemical called *acetaldehyde* and is later converted to acetate by an enzyme called *acetaldehyde dehydrogenase.* Some populations have an underactive form of acetaldehyde dehydrogenase that results in the rapid buildup of acetaldehyde if too much alcohol is consumed. Increased levels of acetaldehyde cause the face to turn hot and scarlet, intense throbbing is felt in the head and neck, and a severe headache develops. It may be expected that such individuals will tend to avoid using alcohol to any great extent. These interethnic differences in drug response often have a genetic basis that suggests drug use may have evolutionary consequences.

Liver enzyme alleles most often account for population differences in drug sensitivity. This is because the liver is the primary internal organ that metabolizes drugs. Within the cells of the liver there exists a large group of enzymes technically known as the *cytochrome P450* system. This enzyme system plays an important role in the initial steps of drug metabolism. Approximately 600 cytochrome P450 genes have been described—some of their alleles have significant effects on the rate at which drugs are metabolized. The cytochrome P450 enzyme encoded by a gene called *CYP2D6* provides an interesting example. One allele causes a loss of enzyme function and a significantly impaired ability to metabolize drugs, such as antidepressants or amphetamines. By contrast, other individuals are "ultrarapid metabolizers" because they have several copies of the CYP2D6 gene. In some cases this CYP2D6 gene has been duplicated up to a dozen times. This results in the production of many copies of the enzyme protein with the consequence of more rapid drug breakdown and elimination. In other words, a greater amount of drug is required to achieve the same effect as in individuals who lack duplicated copies of the gene.

There is also evidence that certain alleles of drug metabolizing enzymes have grown more frequent in particular human populations. Over time, these gene alleles seem to have been selected in an evolutionary manner. This would imply that they confer some advantage on the population that carries the allele. The cytochrome P450 system provides yet another example. An allele of the CYP2D6 gene, denoted *CYP2D*4*, is common in Caucasian (white) populations but virtually absent in Asian, Native American, and some

African (Ethiopian and Zimbabwean) populations. One explanation for this difference is that the allele appeared in Caucasians after
their separation from Asian and would-be Native American groups
some 35,000 years ago.

Genetic polymorphism, which refers to the presence of more
than one allele in a population, is not restricted to effects on drug
metabolism—drug receptor alleles also exist. Not all patients who
suffer from schizophrenia respond to treatment with clozapine. The
patients who do respond have an allele of the gene encoding a particular form of the serotonin receptor, which is called *5HT2A*. The
treatment of Alzheimer's disease provides yet another example.
Apolipoprotein E is important blood protein that carries fats, such as
cholesterol and triglycerides, to the fat-storing cells of the body. In
the brain apolipoprotein E seems to play an additional role in maintaining the normal functioning of nerve cells. There are three major
alleles of apolipoprotein E, and the one denoted *apoE4* is indicative
of a risk of the early onset of Alzheimer's disease. Individuals who
carry the apoE4 allele respond favorably to tacrine, a drug that
enhances the action of the acetylcholine neurotransmitter by blocking the enzyme that inactivates it.

Our understanding of human genetic polymorphism is still in
its infancy. Many more alleles for drug receptors and their metabolizing enzymes are likely to be identified. Presumably, the persistence of these alleles over many generations confers some advantage
to the individuals of the population that carry it. In many respects
the evolution of our genome has been drug driven.

Plant Symbiosis

About a quarter of all prescriptions are for drugs that contain compounds originally identified in plants, fungi, or various microorganisms. Taxol (paclitaxel, an anticancer drug), morphine, digoxin,
and penicillin are but a few examples. We have coevolved with these

plants and fungi and, in many instances, deliberately modified their characteristics for our benefit. The development of our cereal crops involved the painstaking domestication of wild grasses through the selection of varieties with larger and less bitter seeds. The selection of cannabis plant varieties for a higher content of psychoactive cannabinoids is another, more recent, example.

Plants have the amazing ability to synthesize the most complex chemicals. Our bodies cannot synthezise benzodiazepines—their structure is far too complex. Yet benzodiazepines have been found in human brains preserved in blocks of paraffin, since the mid-1940s, long before the chemist Leo Sternbach at the Roche drug company had identified them. They are found, too, in the brains of cattle, in quantities sufficient to have a significant biological effect. Benzodiazepines are also found in laboratory animals. This reduces the possibility that their source is an industrially synthesized drug because laboratory animals are maintained on a controlled diet and in a restricted environment.

A possible source of our brain benzodiazepines may be plants. It appears that some plants can synthesize part of the benzodiazepine molecule and that certain microorganisms can complete the process. Forage, such as grasses of the *Festuca* species or clover of the *Trifolium* species, do not contain detectable amounts of benzodi-azepines, nor does the bovine rumen. But a four-hour incubation of this forage with rumen micro-rganisms results in the rapid syn-thesis of benzodiazepine-like molecules that have exactly the same properties as benzodiazepines synthesized in the laboratory. This would explain why benzodiazepines are found in milk and the blood of individuals who have never knowingly consumed them.

Archaeologists inform us that the switch to an agrarian lifestyle, previously dubbed the Neolithic Revolution, was more of a slow and complex evolution in which hunter-gatherers first settled in small communities experimenting with the cultivation of cereals, some 13,000 years ago. For centuries they continued to hunt wild game, only later becoming full-fledged farmers living in populous villages with domesticated plants and animals. Such societies then raised more children to adulthood, enjoyed food surpluses, clustered in villages, and set off down the road to build the great cities of civilization. This novel way of life diffused across the world. Did their brain "benzodiazepines" reduce anxiety and facilitate the structuring of these close-knit communities? Many more psychoactive substances are likely to be synthesised by the plants with which we have coevolved.

But why do plants produce psychoactive substances? One possibility is that these chemicals provide the plant with some protection from insect predators. Caffeine, for example, is a bitter substance, which may prevent insects from eating more plants that contain a high content of the chemical. Alternatively, the action of substances such as nicotine, morphine, or tetrahydrocannabinol may have such a profound effect on the nervous system of the insect that it becomes completely disoriented and cannot feed further on the plant. However, tea, coffee, and tobacco farmers still need to rely heavily on the use of insecticides to protect their crops, so the chemicals-as-defense theory cannot be the entire explanation for the presence of so many psychoactive substances in different kinds of plants. Another possibility for the existence of psychoactive substances in plants is that they regulate cell-to-cell communication. Nicotine, morphine, caffeine, and tetrahydrocannabinol act at brain receptors to modulate cell-to-cell signaling. It is not unreasonable to assume that they may play a similar role in plants.

Traditionally, the electrical impulse has been regarded as the defining functional property of nerve cells; after all, it is the only means by which signals can be effectively delivered over the great distances covered by nerve cell axons. But skeletal muscle and cardiac cells can also generate electrical impulses. Even a simple, single-cell organism, like *Paramecium*, uses electrical impulses to control the propelling action of hair-like structures, called *cilia*, on its surface. It should not be surprising, therefore, that long-stemmed plants, such as peas, use electrical impulses to move the sap through their vessels. And when an insect triggers the Venus fly trap, electrical impulses cause the leaves to close rapidly on its prey.

Plants also contain many chemicals that can act as agonists at brain glutamate receptors and, therefore, have the potential to alter memory processes, such as those exemplified by LTP. Examples include quisqualic acid found in the seeds of a liana known as the Rangoon creeper (*Quisqualis indica*) and kainic acid synthesized by the seaweed *Digenea simplex*. Plant glutamate agonists are abundant, but the existence of glutamate receptors in plants is really surprising. These receptors are not unlike those of the brain. They are found in all sorts of plants, including maize, rice, tobacco, and pea, where they appear to play a functional role. When a seedling such as *Arabidopsis*, a member of the cabbage family, is grown on agar containing a specific glutamate receptor antagonist, its ability to produce chlorophyll in response to light is significantly impaired. Chemical signaling at the glutamate receptor, therefore, is a basic requirement for plants, since chlorophyll is essential for the production of energy by the process of photosynthesis. It is likely that many other receptor types, at which psychoactive chemicals mediate a physiological response, will be identified in plants.

But excessive exposure to many of these plant glutamate agonists may cause degeneration of nerve cells. In experimental models such agonists have been found to be capable of literally stimulating a cell to death. Nicotine is also toxic. An ordinary cigar contains enough nicotine, about sixty milligrams, to kill two mice. The burning of the tobacco, however, destroys much of the nicotine, and it is subsequently poorly absorbed into the bloodstream when chewed or swallowed. Generally speaking, we have learned to enjoy and survive these plant chemicals, presumably, as a result of fortuitous mutations in neurotransmitter receptors involved in their actions or in the enzyme proteins that detoxify them.

The Icon of Our Era

The historical milestones of pharmacology have been described, as well as the way in which drugs may physically sculpt memory to drive the evolution of society. But the future of pharmacology may be based on our genes. The Human Genome Project was established in 1990. The goal of the Project is to work out the complete DNA sequence of the human genome, in essence, to describe all 80–100,000 human genes. The project is almost complete. Biology, medicine, and industry have forged a powerful alliance in one of the biggest initiatives ever undertaken by science. It will reframe our concepts of disease and therapy forever.

One potential outcome from the Human Genome Project could be the ultimate achievement of specific medical therapy, the manipulation of our genes, the very stuff of life itself. A major driving force of the Project is the identification of genes that predispose us to disease in order that they may be "cured" by gene therapy; that is, physically replace the defective gene with a normal one. But promises of replacing damaged genes have been with us for more than a decade without any unequivocal case of successful gene therapy. Moreover, there now exists a growing divergence of opinion among scientists as to whether it is possible that the function of a single gene can either cause or cure a disease. Indeed, it is very difficult to predict the role of genes in any complex biological function. Huntington's disease, for example, is a relatively rare brain disorder associated with symptoms of depression, personality change, impaired memory, and abnormal involuntary movements. It results from the inheritance of a single abnormal gene, which encodes a protein called *huntingtin* of unknown function. An important feature of Huntington's disease is that it does not strike until middle age, which illustrates the critical point that a particular gene, although transmitted at conception, may exert no detectable influence for many years. Moreover, the abnormal form of huntingtin is rarely found in the neurons most vulnerable to the disease. Why the same gene can be present in many different kinds of cells but only some be affected is not known. The interaction of some other gene(s) must be required.

Is it wrong to believe that understanding everything about a single gene will allow us to predict both its normal and abnormal functioning in the body? The question encapsulates the current dilemma because it challenges the role of both genes and the scientific method. This debate has brought matters of health and science closer to the center of public consciousness than ever before. Gone are the days when we put our faith in the goodwill of the healer. Social, moral, ethical, and financial issues now have to be considered. Genetic screening may invade our privacy, increase the cost of our insurance policies, confer the death sentence on a malformed infant, or lead to the release of a serial killer from Death Row. Little did German Nobel Prize-winner Max Delbrück and his coterie of physicists who founded the new discipline of molecular biology realize that their heirs would face some of the same moral and ethical issues they faced when they gave us the atom bomb.

Yet the identification of every single gene and, by extrapolation, the structure of the proteins they encode has great potential for the pharmacologist, because it will allow the development of drugs with unique specificity on a scale never before imagined. The flow of gene information from the Human Genome Project is so massive that our existing knowledge base will have to be buttressed by the emerging science of bioinformatics and combinatorial chemistry. These techniques allow us to sift through databases to compare, contrast, and continually modify a basic chemical structure until the perfect fit for its target receptor is achieved. The limits to drug development are now conceptual, not technological. The time has come again when science must reshape its therapies for the future. This time we are aware of the choices and consequences.

What the future seems to hold is an array of synthetic drugs that will precisely alter brain function. If the pharmacologist is in charge of designing the product, the physician will in turn become an engineer who adapts the new technology to the needs and desires of the individual. Balancing molecules and case histories, the physician will mediate between new products and the idiosyncrasies of the patient. Pharmacology and its psychiatric translations are about to emerge in a flurry of excitement and importance, analogous to those previously associated with particle physics and presently with the new genetics. This creates the impression that the days of humanistic psychology are gone and that the new age will be heralded by philosophical and legalistic debate about our use of drugs in the future. The era of the shaman is over.

Further Readings

Bahn, Paul G. *Prehistoric Art*. New York: Cambridge University Press, 1998.

Barondes, Samuel. *Molecules and Mental Illness*. New York: Scientific American Library, W. H. Freeman and Company, 1993.

Bear, Mark F., Barry W. Connors, and Michael A. Paradiso. *Neuroscience: Exploring the Brain*. Baltimore, Md.: Williams and Wilkins, 1996.

Braun, Stephen. *Buzz: The Science and Lore of Alcohol and Caffeine*. New York: Oxford University Press, 1996.

Cavalli-Sforza, L. Luca, Paolo Menozzi, and Alberto Piazza. *The History and Geography of Human Genes*, abridged edition. Princeton, N.J.: Princeton University Press, 1996.

Connerton, Paul. *How Societies Remember*. New York: Cambridge University Press, 1989.

Crick, Francis. *The Astonishing Hypothesis: The Scientific Search for the Soul*. New York: Simon and Schuster, 1994.

Drews, Jürgen. *In Quest of Tomorrow's Medicines*. New York: Springer-Verlag, 1999.

Feldman, Robert S., Jerrold S. Meyer, and Linda F. Quenzer. *Principles of Neuropsychopharmacology*. Sunderland, Mass.: Sinauer Associates, 1997.

Finger, Stanley. *Origins of Neuroscience: A History of Explorations Into Brain Function*. New York: Oxford University Press, 1994.

Foucault, Michel. *Madness and Civilization: A History of Insanity in the Age of Reason*. London: Routledge, 1967.

Grilly, Daniel M. *Drugs and Human Behaviour*. Third edition. Needham Heights, Mass.: Allyn and Bacon, 1998.

Healy, David. *The Anti-Depressant Era*. Cambridge, Mass.: Harvard University Press, 1997.

Iversen, Leslie L. *The Science of Marijuana*. New York: Oxford University Press, 2000.

Kutchins, Herb and Stuart A. Kirk. *Making Us Crazy: DSM: The Psychiatric Bible and the Creation of Mental Disorders*. New York: The Free Press, 1997.

LeDoux, Joseph. *The Emotional Brain: The Mysterious Underpinnings of Emotional Life*. New York: Simon and Schuster, 1996.

Lenson, David. *On Drugs*. Minneapolis, Minn.: University of Minnesota Press, 1995.

Mann, John. *Murder, Magic, and Medicine*. New York: Oxford University Press, 1992.

Michel, George F. and Celia L. Moore. *Developmental Psychobiology: An Interdisciplinary Science*. Cambridge, Mass.: Massachusetts Institute of Technology Press, 1995.

Ott, Jonathan. *Pharmacotheon: Entheogenic Drugs, Their Plant Sources, and History*. Second edition. Kennewick, Wash.: Natural Products Company, 1996.

Rudgley, Richard. *The Alchemy of Culture: Intoxicants in Society*. London: British Museum Press, 1993.

Schildkraut, Joseph J. and Aurora Otera, eds. *Depression and the Spiritual in Modern Art: Homage to Miró*. New York: John Wiley and Sons, 1996.

Shapiro, Arthur K. and Elaine Shapiro. *The Powerful Placebo: From Ancient Priest to Modern Physician*. Baltimore, Md.: Johns Hopkins University Press, 1997.

Shepherd, Gordon M. *Neurobiology*. Third edition. New York: Oxford University Press, 1994.

Snyder, Solomon. *Drugs and the Brain.* New York: Scientific American Library, W. H. Freeman and Company, 1986.

Sonnedecker, Glenn. *Kremers and Urdang's History of Pharmacy.* Revised fourth edition. Madison, Wis.: J. B. Lippincott Company, 1976.

Stearns, Stephen C., ed. *Evolution in Health and Disease.* New York: Oxford University Press, 1999.

Squire, Larry R. *Memory and Brain.* New York: Oxford University Press, 1987.

Squire, Larry R. and Eric R. Kandel. *Memory: From Mind to Molecules.* New York: Scientific American Library, W. H. Freeman and Company, 1999.

United Nations International Drug Control Programme. *World Drug Report.* New York: Oxford University Press, 1997.

Young, John Z. *Philosophy and the Brain.* New York: Oxford University Press, 1987.

Index